cl

OXFORD MEDICAL PUBLICATIONS

Cystic Fibrosis

THE FACTS

cl

ALSO PUBLISHED BY OXFORD UNIVERSITY PRESS

Ageing: the facts
(second edition)
Nicholas Coni, William Davison,
and Stephen Webster

Alcoholism: the facts
(second edition)
Donald W. Goodwin

Allergy: the facts
Robert J. Davies and
Susan Ollier

**Arthritis and rheumatism:
the facts** (second edition)
J. T. Scott

Autism: the facts
Simon Baron-Cohen and
Patrick Bolton

Back pain: the facts
(third edition)
Malcolm I. V. Jayson

Bowel cancer: the facts
John M. A. Northover and
Joel D. Kettner

Childhood leukaemia: the facts
John S. Lilleyman

Contraception: the facts
(second edition)
Peter Bromwich and
Tony Parsons

**Coronary heart disease:
the facts** (second edition)
Desmond Julian and
Claire Marley

Cystic fibrosis: the facts
(third edition)
Ann Harris and Maurice Super

Deafness: the facts
Andrew P. Freeland

**Dyslexia and other learning
difficulties: the facts**
Mark Selikowitz

Eating disorders: the facts
(third edition) Suzanne Abraham
and Derek Llewellyn-Jones

Eczema in childhood: the facts
David J. Atherton

Head injury: the facts
Dorothy Gronwall, Philip
Wrightson, and Peter Waddell

Healthy skin: the facts
Rona M. MacKie

**Liver disease and gallstones:
the facts** (second edition)
Alan G. Johnson and
David R. Triger

Lung cancer: the facts
(second edition)
Chris Williams

Multiple sclerosis: the facts
(third edition)
Bryan Matthews

Muscular dystrophy: the facts
Alan E. H. Emery

**Obsessive–compulsive disorder:
the facts**
Padmal de Silva and
Stanley Rachman

Parkinson's disease: the facts
(second edition)
Gerald Stern and Andrew Lees

Thyroid disease: the facts
(second edition) R. I. S. Bayliss
and W. M. G. Tunbridge

Cystic Fibrosis

THE FACTS
Third Edition

ANN HARRIS

Lecturer in Paediatric Molecular Genetics
Institute of Molecular Medicine, University of Oxford

and

MAURICE SUPER

Consultant Paediatric Geneticist, Royal
Manchester Children's Hospital

Oxford   New York   Tokyo
OXFORD UNIVERSITY PRESS
1995

Oxford University Press, Walton Street, Oxford OX2 6DP

Oxford New York
Athens Auckland Bangkok Bombay
Calcutta Cape Town Dar es Salaam Delhi
Florence Hong Kong Istanbul Karachi
Kuala Lumpur Madras Madrid Melbourne
Mexico City Nairobi Paris Singapore
Taipei Tokyo Toronto
and associated companies in
Berlin Ibadan

Oxford is a trade mark of Oxford University Press

Published in the United States
by Oxford University Press Inc., New York

A catalogue record for this book is available from the British Library

Library of Congress Cataloging in Publication Data
Harris, Ann, 1956–
Cystic fibrosis : the facts / Ann Harris and Maurice Super. — 3rd ed.
(Oxford medical publications) (Facts (Oxford. England))
Includes index.
1. Cystic fibrosis in children—Popular works. I. Super, Maurice.
II. Title. III. Series. IV. Series: Facts (Oxford, England)
RJ456.C9H37 1995 616.3'7—dc20 94-36967
ISBN 0 19 262543 8

Typeset by Downdell, Oxford
Printed in Great Britain by
Biddles Ltd
Guildford & King's Lynn

Preface to the third edition

Publication of the second edition of *Cystic fibrosis—the facts* came shortly after the isolation of the gene for cystic fibrosis at a time of great optimism. Much of that optimism was well founded, with our increased understanding of what the protein that is made by the CFTR gene actually does and how errors in it actually cause the disease. It is now possible to detect defects in the CFTR gene in the vast majority of affected individuals, though in general this does not enable us to predict the severity of disease that will result. The next phase of CF research is now well under way, that is an attempt to correct the basic defect in the disease. At this stage it is impossible to predict whether this will be effective and how long it will be before we will know the outcome. This edition of the book contains a substantially updated approach to living with cystic fibrosis and to the treatment of the disease. It also includes new chapters on genetics and on new treatments.

Oxford
Manchester
February 1995

A.H.
M.S.

Acknowledgements

The authors would like to thank Miss Despina Savva for help with preparation of the original figures. Also John Bateman and Jonathan Super for their respective photographic contributions. We are grateful to Drs Sonja Gatzanis and Margaret Hodson, Mrs Jan Davis, Clive Sandercock, and the late Gary Gifford for helpful discussions and critical reading of parts of the manuscript.

Figure 11 was kindly provided by the cytogenetics department of the Paediatric Research Unit, Division of Medical and Molecular Genetics, UMDS—Guy's Hospital, London.

A.H. would like to thank Professor Paul E. Polani, who introduced her to the subject; and Dr Anne Thomson for her helpful advice.

M.S. thanks Dr Garry Hambleton and the CF team, Royal Manchester Children's Hospital, for helpful discussions.

Contents

1 What is cystic fibrosis?

Cystic fibrosis is an inherited disease that has its main effects on the digestive system and the lungs. It is usually diagnosed soon after birth, and symptoms occur throughout life. Nowadays, thanks to improvements in dietary supplements and better treatment, most people with cystic fibrosis can lead a fairly normal life. However, to achieve this they need daily treatment, consisting of chest physiotherapy, various medicines, and pancreatic enzyme capsules taken with their food. In addition they have to pay special attention to their increased dietary needs.

The name cystic fibrosis (CF) describes the changes that occur at an early age in the pancreas of CF patients. (The pancreas is a major organ in the body, manufacturing digestive enzymes and other important compounds.) The part of the pancreas that produces digestive enzymes (proteins that digest food) is replaced by characteristic fibrous scar tissue with fluid-filled spaces (cysts).

Another common feature of CF is unusually sticky or thick mucus secretions in the lungs and digestive system. In the lungs the presence of this thick or viscid mucus makes chest infections more severe. In the digestive system it may damage the pancreas, both directly and indirectly, by blocking the ducts that would usually form an open channel for digestive enzymes to reach the gut. This viscid mucus is the origin of another common name for CF: mucoviscidosis.

Until the beginning of this century doctors did not recognize CF as a disease in its own right. The various symptoms of CF were merely seen as separate, unrelated infections. Part of the reason for this was that before the advent of antibiotics, chest infections (which are a major feature of CF) were common in many diseases. The first recognition of CF came through another feature of the disease, namely steatorrhoea. Steatorrhoea means literally 'fatty stools', and is a condition characterized by the passage of pale, bulky, smelly faeces. Thus in 1912 the London physician Archibald Garrod described the occurrence of steatorrhoea in several members

of the same family. The description, with hindsight, was almos
certainly of CF.

The next clear description of CF came from a Swiss paediatrician
named Fanconi. He described children with cystic fibrosis in 1928
and again in 1936. He also distinguished CF from coeliac disease, a
disease caused by an inability to digest wheat proteins that ha
some symptoms in common with CF. When the initial description
of CF were made, there was some controversy as to whether steato
rrhoea and recurrent attacks of severe bronchitis constituted a
separate disease (both symptoms were common to several disease
in the pre-antibiotic era). It was not until other chest and digestiv
system diseases (for example pneumonia and bacillary dysentery
became treatable that this controversy was resolved.

It was found that in some cases treatment of chest or gut infec
tions was ineffective, or gave only temporary relief. The patient
unaffected by treatment were identified as CF sufferers. Thu
Fanconi, working in Zurich, and Dorothy Anderson in Baltimore
were proved correct in recognizing CF as a specific disorder
A paper by Dorothy Anderson in 1938 gave an almost complete
account of the development of CF, and a further paper in 1946 ad
vocated treatment of the disease with a high-calorie, high-protein
low-fat diet supplemented with pancreatin (extract of anima
pancreas). In 1948 Anderson and her coworker Di'Santagnese
confirmed another characteristic of the disease. They showed tha
CF patients are particularly prone to chest infections caused by
Staphylococcus bacteria.

In 1952 there was a heatwave in New York. Perceptive physician
noted that the majority of children brought to casualty department
with heat prostration were CF sufferers. This led Di'Santagnese to
the discovery of the greatly increased levels of salt in the sweat o
people with CF. This has become the cornerstone on which the
diagnosis of CF rests. Parents may notice a salty taste when they
kiss their CF baby. Two physiologists, Gibson and Cooke, realized
the need for a standard technique for collecting sweat for testing
and described a method of stimulating sweat production and
collecting it.

One of the symptoms considered as an almost certain sign of CF
was, in fact, first described in 1905 by Landsteiner. In translation

the title of his article reads: 'Intestinal obstruction from thickened meconium'. The first dark-green stools passed after birth are called meconium, and meconium ileus (an obstruction of the small intestine) affects 10–15 per cent of those infants destined to show the other signs of CF.

Poor absorption of food is a characteristic of most people with CF who go untreated. It manifests itself as steatorrhoea (non-digestion of fat leading to bulky, strong-smelling stools). There are also a number of other ways in which the disease may show its presence. In infants, the steatorrhoea may be accompanied by prolapse of the rectum (a condition where the very frequent passage of bulky stools causes the lining of the rectum to protrude through the anus). The first symptoms of CF in the young child are often confused with milk allergy.

Cystic fibrosis sufferers are also subject to recurrent chest infections. These are caused by bacteria, notably *Staphylococcus aureus*, the different types of *Pseudomonas*, and *Haemophilus influenzae*. While *Staphylococcus aureus* is an aggressive bacterium that causes disease in healthy people, *Pseudomonas* is an opportunist, that requires a weakness in the tissue it is attacking before it can gain a foothold. Conditions in the lungs of CF patients provide the right environment for these organisms to thrive and generally, although not always, one or other organism is found. Before antistaphylococcal antibiotics were discovered, *Staphylococcus aureus* predominated. The effects of repeated chest infections usually led to death by seven years of age. Now, survival is much longer and a progression from staphylococcal to pseudomonal infection is common in those patients more severely affected.

As suggested above, there is great variation in the severity of CF, even within members of the same family. A number of studies have shown that girls with CF generally do slightly worse than boys. Nevertheless, a good number of affected girls have grown up to have children. The vast majority of men with CF are sterile; Shwachman showed in 1968 that this was due to fibrosis of the epididymis and absence of a vas deferens. These two ducts normally form a conduit through which sperm pass on their way from the testis to the exterior of the body.

Puberty used to be delayed in CF but with better nutrition this problem arises much less frequently. When inadequate weight gain does occur in CF this is often in adolescence, a time when normal adolescent rebellion can result in resistance to physiotherapy and the taking of medicines, including pancreatic enzymes.

Cystic fibrosis is a hereditary disease. Cedric Carter, in 1952, was the first to recognize the way in which the CF gene is transmitted from one generation to the next. The disease is caused by a pair of abnormal *recessive* genes in each cell of the body (a gene is a small portion of the genetic material, that is concerned with the making of a protein). The effects of a single recessive gene are masked when the normal form of the same gene also occurs in the same cell in a carrier. The defective gene in CF is on an autosome, the disease occurring equally often in males and females (this is discussed further in Chapter 7). The illness CF affects only those individuals who have inherited the defective gene from *both* their mother and father. If two carriers marry there is a one in four chance that any of their children may inherit the gene from each of them. No adverse health problems occur for the parents through being carriers.

Cystic fibrosis is the commonest autosomal recessive genetic disease of white Indo-Europeans (Caucasians). In most parts of the world, between 1 in 1500 and 1 in 2500 Caucasian children are born with CF, though the disease may not be apparent at birth. If one takes these two sets of frequencies then between 1 in 16 and 1 in 25 Caucasians is a carrier.

On average, one child with CF is born every day in the United Kingdom, and four to five daily in the United States. In fact, the condition occurs wherever Europeans have settled. It is extremely rare in the Chinese and in the Negro races in Africa. In some Third World countries, with high infant mortality, a diagnosis of CF could easily be missed. In Britain, we do see CF in children of Pakistani and Arab descent. The incidence in their countries of origin is unknown.

Until recently there was no reliable test to detect a CF carrier, and carrier status could only be established after the birth of a CF child to a particular couple. Over the last couple of years, research advances have dramatically altered this situation. In many cases we can now tell if a person drawn at random from the general population carries a defective CF gene, by directly testing his or her genetic material. In other words, that person does not have to produce a CF child before we know that he or she carries a CF gene. Precisely how this test is done will be explained more fully in Chapter 7. The people who have demonstrated most interest in knowing their carrier status are the relatives of those with CF and their partners.

Late in 1985, it was established by research groups in Denmark, Canada, America, and England that the gene causing CF was located on chromosome 7. Nearly four years later, in September 1989, a tremendous research effort from several large groups of scientists culminated in the publication, in the American journal *Science*, of the isolation of the CF gene itself. Collaborating research groups in Canada and North America had finally achieved the feat that the CF world had been awaiting for so long. However, it should be remembered that this is really only the beginning of the story in terms of understanding how the CF gene acts to cause the disease. In the piece of genetic information that is the CF gene, research scientists now have the tool to start asking fundamental questions about the disease process in CF and how more effective treatments might be developed.

Despite the lack of information on the basic defect, an aggressive approach to treatment has resulted in increased survival and improved health for CF sufferers. Time out of school or off work has been reduced through better attention to chest infections, a positive attitude to chest physiotherapy, adequate dietary intake, and early recognition of danger signs. Treatment is best coordinated in a multidisciplinary CF clinic and is mostly on an out-patient basis. Certain treatments have not stood the test of time. Notable among these is the use of mist tents, in which affected children used to sleep, and special low-fat diets. We continue to search for effective treatments and to question the necessity of treatments that involve sacrifice of time or convenience by the affected person or their family. Unfortunately, many of the effective treatments still do require such sacrifice.

Over the past 10–20 years there has been a gradual but significant improvement in the life expectancy of CF patients, due to

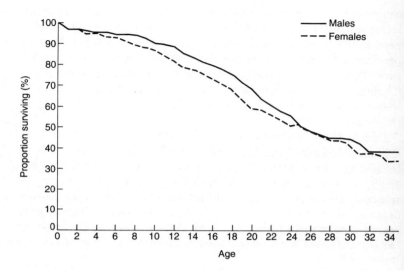

Figure 1 Cystic fibrosis—current survival. (Figures kindly provided by UK CF survey and reproduced with permission.)

advances in the efficacy of treatment. Current predictions of life expectancy suggest that a child born this year with CF is likely to have a median life expectancy of 40 years (see Figure 1). However, it should be mentioned that this is an average figure and, regrettably, some babies will continue to die from CF as will children of all ages and young adults.

There is controversy about some aspects of CF treatment. In the long term, it is hoped that the discovery of the CF gene will enable aspects of treatment to become simpler, more directly aimed at correcting the basic defect in the disease and so less controversial. In writing a book on 'the facts' we have tried hard to be objective and to highlight the more readily acceptable points.

2 Living with cystic fibrosis

Andrew, now aged 14, was diagnosed as having cystic fibrosis when he was two years old. He has recently had a button gastrostomy inserted because of persistently poor weight gain. He is an intelligent boy with a fertile imagination. These are his unedited comments.

I first realized that I was different when I went to school. I would get out of breath when playing with my friends, and start coughing up thick mucus. My parents would pat me on my back and my sides to help clear my chest of mucus every day before I went to school and every evening before I went to bed. I sometimes found myself in an ambulance and being pricked with needles.

I look on CF as a challenge, not to let myself get depressed and upset because I am a bit different. I make sure that I have all my medication and treatment on a regular basis. Sometimes I find this difficult, being surrounded by people who lead normal lives, and don't have medication or go to hospital. My brothers make this hard to accept, both being bigger and stronger than me (Andrew has a twin and an older brother). They try to make me something I am not and probably never will be.

I sometimes get embarrassed when people see me taking a lot of tablets, looking at me as if I was a drug addict. I used to get called 'mobile chemist' or 'druggie', which got on my nerves a lot.

I am very optimistic about genetic engineering, although apprehensive too.

In my spare time I do various activities. I am a member of the Air Training Corps and also play in the band. I have recently been awarded 'Trumpeter of the Year' in my squadron, and I am now learning to play the baritone—all good exercise for the lungs! I am looking forward to going on the adventure camp weekends and gaining my bronze Duke of Edinburgh Award. Our squadron also competes in sporting activities, so I get plenty of exercise.

I know my CF will not go away and I can't ignore it, but I have to get on with my life and enjoy it. So I hope people will know me as Andrew, and not 'that boy with CF'. CF is just part of me, just the same as the colour of my eyes and hair. **It's just me.**

The following are comments from the mother of a CF child, Sarah, who is now aged six. She was diagnosed at the age of one year, at which time she already had a collapsed right upper lobe of her lung. At three years she had a lobectomy, since which she has remained fairly well.

When my daughter was first diagnosed as having CF, I suppose I became a blubbering wreck. To be told that Sarah, who we thought was a perfectly healthy baby, had an inherited gene disorder which we had unknowingly passed on to her and which, unlike other childhood illnesses, she would never grow out of, was very hard to adjust to.

After diagnosis, a strict regime of physiotherapy, morning and evening, fell into place. My daughter now had to take countless pills and potions, making my medicine cupboard look like a chemist's shop. There were also many out-patients' appointments and a few stays in hospital as the years passed.

Having a child with CF means that you are on a constant roller-coaster of highs and lows. It is great when they are well, as life is able to follow some sort of normality, but when they become ill (which can happen very quickly) you hit the all-time lows and the 'if onlies' spring to mind.

I have always been of the opinion that Sarah should be treated exactly the same as any other child of her age. She participates in all aspects of physical activity at school and though she is not the best sports person in the world, I emphasize that sport is good for her and, after all, it is the taking part that matters.

Over the years we have experienced the rebellious stages: hating 50 minutes of physio (she used to hide under the bed); not wanting to take her tablets (a minimum of 60 per day); and at one stage refusing to use the nebulizer, although eventually all these problems were overcome.

Having a child with CF (as well as two non-CF children) means that my days have to be well planned, enabling me to cater for everyone's needs and, most importantly, to make sure that Sarah still gets the care she requires to remain as fit and healthy as possible.

3 What is happening in the body in cystic fibrosis?

Three main systems in the body are classically affected by cystic fibrosis. These are the lungs and respiratory tract, the digestive system (particularly the pancreas and intestines), and the sweat glands. In this chapter the effects of CF on each of these three systems will be discussed in more detail.

The lungs and respiratory tract

Figure 2 shows the normal anatomy of the respiratory tree. Air enters the nostrils and the nasal sinuses, then passes into the single tube of the trachea or windpipe. The trachea splits at its bottom end into two bronchi (one for each lung), and the bronchi continue to divide into smaller and smaller tubes (bronchioles), ending in thousands of small air sacs (alveoli). It is from the alveoli that oxygen enters the bloodstream and carbon dioxide is released.

From the upper airways down to the bronchioles, the respiratory tree is lined with many small, hair-like protrusions called cilia. The cilia are covered in a thin layer of mucus. They beat in a wave-like motion to waft the mucus and any extraneous matter (including bacteria) towards the nose or pharynx. Whatever reaches the upper part of the respiratory tree is either swallowed or coughed out. Ciliary action will normally act against gravity to clear the various lobes of the lung, whatever position the body may be in.

In CF, however, mucus tends to clog up the upper and lower respiratory tree. It is possible that as a secondary effect of the basic defect in CF the mucous secretions contain less water than they should. It is clear from detailed research that poor mucus clearance is not due to uneven ciliary beating (the synchronized beating of cilia lining the respiratory tree normally wafts mucus upwards and

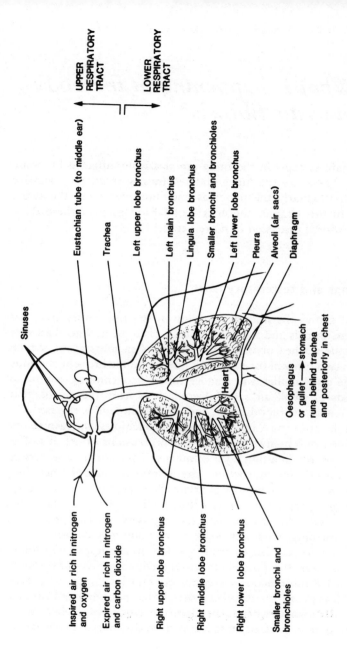

Figure 2 Diagram of the human respiratory tree.

Inspired air rich in nitrogen and oxygen

Expired air rich in nitrogen and carbon dioxide

Right upper lobe bronchus

Right middle lobe bronchus

Right lower lobe bronchus

Smaller bronchi and bronchioles

Sinuses

Eustachian tube (to middle ear)

Trachea

Left upper lobe bronchus

Left main bronchus

Lingula lobe bronchus

Smaller bronchi and bronchioles

Left lower lobe bronchus

Pleura

Alveoli (air sacs)

Diaphragm

Heart

Oesophagus or gullet → stomach runs behind trachea and posteriorly in chest

UPPER RESPIRATORY TRACT

LOWER RESPIRATORY TRACT

out of the lungs). However, there is no doubt that mucus is poorly cleared against gravity in the presence of bacterial infection.

Build-up of mucus in the lungs can have several consequences. Ball-valve effects occur in those segments of the lung that have become overdistended because air passes an obstruction on breathing in, but does not all pass back on breathing out. These obstructions are caused by mucus and airway narrowing. The overinflation becomes more marked with time, and results in emphysema, a state of overdistension in which the elasticity of the lung is reduced. Deformity of the chest develops, with rounding of the shoulders and prominence of the sternum. Occasionally, and usually late in the course of the disease, distended alveoli at the surface of the lung may rupture, giving rise to pneumothorax (air between the surface of the lung and the chest wall) requiring special treatment. This damage is compounded by recurrent or continuous chest infections, or by bronchiectasis, a state of permanent weakening of the bronchial walls and poor drainage of infected mucus. Bronchiectasis is associated with permanent lung infection and clubbing of the fingers. Clubbing occurs as a result of substances associated with the lung infections entering the blood. In some way these stimulate the growth of the soft tissue at the bases of the finger and toenails, causing loss of the angle between the nail and the skin.

Abnormalities in the air and blood supply to the lungs may result from CF. These abnormalities may not be immediately apparent, as the reserve capacity of the lungs allows them to function normally even when quite significantly damaged. Studies with radioactive compounds either injected into a vein or inhaled (see Chapter 4, p. 30, and Fig. 9) can show the extent of the tissue damage.

Bacterial infections in the respiratory tree in CF

Though a number of bacterial chest infections may occur in CF, the commonest is caused by *Staphylococcus aureus*. Infection by an organism causing less damage to the lungs, *Haemophilus influenzae*, may occur intermittently. Later in the course of the disease, infection by *Pseudomonas* bacteria may also occur. *Staphylococcus aureus* is a micro-organism that does not occur in the body naturally, but only as part of an infection. It may cause minor problems such as pimples, or more major ones like osteomyelitis (a bone infection) in the general population, but in CF it is found together with chronic (long-term) bronchitis and lung infection. The bacterium *Pseudomonas aeruginosa* does not infect healthy tissue. It only attacks damaged tissue, for example the skin in severe burns, or the lungs in CF, when a certain degree of damage and loss of some of the healthy lining of the bronchi has occurred. Different varieties of *Pseudomonas* are recognized by their laboratory characteristics. There seem to be two forms of the bacteria, non-mucoid and mucoid. The mucoid type has a slimy appearance and once acquired it is seldom eradicated. Though a cause of less tissue damage than *Staphylococcus*, an established mucoid *Pseudomonas* infection is generally associated with deterioration in lung function. Recently different strains of organisms related to *Pseudomonas aeruginosa* have been found in patients with CF, namely *Pseudomonas cepacia* and *Pseudomonas maltophilia*. Sometimes these are more invasive than the aeruginosa type.

Non-bacterial infection in CF

Older children and adults with CF may show the effects of infection by a fungus, *Aspergillus fumigatus*, which may be found in the sputum and give rise to antifungal antibodies in the blood. Together the fungus and the antibodies may set up an allergic reaction in the lung causing bronchospasm and changes that are detectable on a lung X-ray. Occasionally a ball of fungus called an aspergilloma may grow in the lung cavity.

The upper respiratory tract in CF

Cystic fibrosis may cause changes in the nose and in other parts of the respiratory tree above the trachea. Nasal polyps (protuberant growths of the mucous membranes) develop in the nose in many older children. They occasionally require surgical removal, but have a tendency to recur.

The gastrointestinal tract

The effects of CF on the gastrointestinal tract are numerous and complex. To help understand them more fully, an outline of the normal process of digestion and metabolism of food is given below.

Introduction to digestion and metabolism

In the normal digestive process, food is broken down both mechanically (by chewing) and chemically from complex molecules such as proteins, fats, and carbohydrates (starch) to smaller, simpler molecules such as amino acids, fatty acids, and sugars. This allows food to be absorbed into the body through the walls of the small intestine or ileum (see Figure 3), and then transported in the blood to the liver. The liver is the central chemical factory of the body: here the amino acids and other small molecules are used as building blocks for the body's own proteins, carbohydrates, etc. These then circulate in the bloodstream and are taken up by the various body tissues (for example the lungs, muscles, brain, etc.) as they need them. Tissues need a constant supply of proteins and other nutrients because many cells live only a few days or weeks and there is a constant replacement of dead or dying cells.

Let us look briefly at the individual food types and their fates.

Proteins Proteins are made of long chains of amino acids, coiled into complex shapes. In the digestive system they are broken down first into peptides (short amino acid chains), then to individual amino acids. Proteins serve many functions in the body. They are essential for tissue growth and repair, and enzymes (the molecules that speed up and control the many thousands of chemical reactions in the body) are proteins. In long-term infections or diseases like CF, large amounts of protein are needed for constant tissue repair, and even a high-protein diet may not supply enough for the body's needs.

Fats Fats and oils are broken down in the digestive system to glycerol and fatty acids. Fats are important for energy storage: for

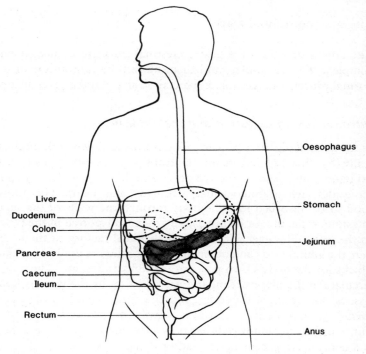

Figure 3 Diagram of the human digestive system.

this they are deposited under the skin in what is known as sub-cutaneous fat. Other functions of fats are as lubricants and in the formation of cell membranes.

Carbohydrates (starch) Carbohydrates are long, branched and unbranched chains of polysaccharides. They are broken down to shorter chains, and thence to disaccharides such as sucrose, maltose, and lactose. These disaccharides are then split into their component monosaccharides (e.g. glucose, fructose, galactose). Both mono- and disaccharides are referred to as sugars.

Besides its function in manufacturing proteins, fats, and carbo-hydrates, the liver is responsible for the breakdown and detoxification of waste products in the body. These waste products then pass out of the body in the urine or faeces. The body uses only glucose products in metabolism and so, in the liver, all monosaccharides are converted to glucose compounds. Glucose is the main fuel for the chemical cycle that supplies energy for the body's functions. Ready glucose energy is stored in the liver and muscles as glycogen. When glycogen stores are full, the excess is stored as fat.

The digestive tract   The parts of the digestive tract (see Figure 2) involved in each step of digestion are as follows. In the mouth, food particles are reduced in size by the teeth and the digestion of starch begins with the action of the enzyme amylase present in saliva. The smell and taste of food stimulate the production of saliva and also of gastrin, a hormone (see the Glossary for a definition of a hormone) which acts on the stomach to stimulate the production of enzymes there. After being swallowed, food travels down the oesophagus or gullet to the stomach. (Transport of food through the digestive tract is achieved by the action of muscles in the gut wall.) In the stomach food mixes with hydrochloric acid and the enzyme pepsin (pepsin is responsible for breaking down the protein in the diet to peptides). The food is prevented from leaving the stomach by a valve called the pylorus, which closes off the entrance to the duodenum. The presence of food in the stomach stimulates the production of a hormone called secretin. This hormone travels in the bloodstream to the duodenum, the liver, and the pancreas, where it stimulates the production of digestive juices.

Once the food in the stomach is in the form of a ball, or bolus, the pyloric valve opens and the bolus of food passes into the duodenum. There it encounters an alkaline digestive fluid consisting of bicarbonate, bile, and the enzymes trypsin, amylase, and lipase from the pancreas. Trypsin completes the breaking down of peptides to amino acids. Amylase continues with the breaking down of starch to the disaccharides sucrose, maltose, and lactose. Further enzymes from the walls of the duodenum itself break down the disaccharides to their component monosaccharides. Fats are emulsified by the bile and then broken down by lipase to glycerol and fatty acids.

From the duodenum, the food travels slowly down through the jejunum and ileum. This whole section of the digestive tract is lined with tiny villi, folds in the gut lining, that increase the surface area available for food absorption. Amino acids, monosaccharides, and the smaller fat breakdown products are absorbed into the blood vessels lining the villi and transported from there to the liver. Larger fat breakdown products enter the lymph channels or lacteals. (The lymphatic system, like the blood system, transports materials around the body and helps to defend it from infection.) In the lymph channels the fat particles are coated, rendering them more soluble, before they enter the bloodstream and eventually reach the liver.

Certain substances in the diet that cannot be digested act as dietary fibre, helping to increase the bulk of the bolus and help its passage down the intestinal canal. Notable among these is a poly-saccharide, raffinose, which forms the fibres in many vegetables. The process of digestion continues all the way down to the end of the ileum.

At the end of the ileum, undigested material passes into the caecum, a mixing chamber. From there it enters the colon where much of the water is reabsorbed. Bacteria normally present in the caecum and colon act on the waste products to break them down into faeces by a process of fermentation. The fermentation also results in the formation of gas (flatus or wind). If there is poor absorption of food, especially of fat, this process of fermentation is especially active, and faeces and flatus become foul-smelling. This happens in a person with CF either taking a diet too rich in fat or receiving too little pancreatic supplement. Carbohydrates can also ferment in the intestine, though special forms of carbohydrate such as Polycal® and Hical® are less subject to fermentation. These compounds can be used in CF to increase energy intake without unpleasant side-effects.

The pancreas and CF

As has already been mentioned, one of the major effects of cystic fibrosis is on the pancreas. Replacement of pancreatic cells with fibrous scar tissue begins before birth, and generally gets worse with time. As a result of this tissue damage, caused initially by deposits of dried-up secretions, the pancreas ceases to function properly. Production of pancreatic juices decreases, and as we saw previously this juice contains enzymes essential for the breakdown and absorption of food. In this section we will look in more detail at the function of the pancreas and how it is affected by CF.

The pancreas secretes mainly water, bicarbonate, and protein enzymes. Secretion of pancreatic juices is a continuous process, but the presence of food in the stomach, or certain other stimuli, can increase the rate of secretion. Bicarbonate secreted in the pancreatic juice is essential in changing the pH of the duodenal contents from the acidic stomach pH to the alkaline pH at which pancreatic enzymes function best. (pH is a measure of acidity or alkalinity.) There is some evidence that there is reduced bicarbonate secretion in CF pancreatic juices.

Pancreatic enzymes are responsible for the breakdown of many components of the diet. Brief descriptions of the actions of the three major pancreatic enzymes were given in the previous section. After absorption and entry into the bloodstream these building blocks provide the essential substances for body growth and repair and the fuels on which the body functions.

Malabsorption

As described earlier, when foodstuffs are not adequately digested they cannot be absorbed normally from the intestines. This results in a wide range of symptoms due to abnormal excretion of fat in the faeces (steatorrhoea) and deficiency of vitamins soluble in fat, as well as proteins, minerals, carbohydrates, other vitamins, and water. Steatorrhoea is a major problem in inadequately treated CF. Furthermore, because the fat is only partly digested, it causes irritation of the bowel and this in turn leads to an increase in the frequency and rate of passage of bowel contents.

Deficiency of the enzyme trypsin means that some of the protein in the diet is not fully broken down to amino acids in the duodenum. Some peptide fragments remain, and since these cannot be absorbed, they pass into the lower intestine and bowel. Here they are broken down to amino acids by other enzymes and by bacteria.

As a result, large amounts of amino acids find their way into the faeces, where together with undigested fat they produce a pronounced odour.

The obvious treatment for malabsorption of food is to supplement the levels of natural digestive enzymes. Simultaneously, factors that are lacking from the diet due to abnormal digestion and absorption must be added to the diet in an assimilable form in order to prevent malnutrition. These therapeutic approaches are dealt with in more detail in Chapter 4. Since pancreatic enzymes do not reach the intestine in most cases of CF, pancreatic enzyme supplements are an essential part of treatment. A small percentage of CF patients have normal pancreatic function.

Gastrointestinal symptoms of CF

During the newborn period: meconium ileus   The first stools of a newborn baby are called meconium. Ten to fifteen per cent of the babies with CF have intestinal obstruction in the first few days of life. The small intestine is clogged with sticky meconium, presumably because of thickened mucus from the intestinal glands. This blockage of the lower intestine causes bilious vomiting and swelling of the abdomen. X-rays help to distinguish meconium ileus from other causes of intestinal blockage.

Surgery is generally necessary in meconium ileus, though the administration of hygroscopic (water-attracting) enemas or the use of other substances capable of thinning mucus may occasionally be effective. The most successful operation used to be Bishop and Koop's ileostomy. This entailed bringing a loop of the ileum to open on the abdominal wall. Stools could then be passed above the blockage, while medication could be given through the opening to clear the obstruction (see Figure 4). Once the lower bowel has been unblocked, stools can once again pass along the normal channel. The ileostomy is usually closed 2–3 months later. The immediate prognosis (i.e. chances of recovery) of meconium ileus improved markedly after introduction of the ileostomy operation in the late 1960s.

Care of newborn babies before and after operations has improved greatly in the last ten years. As a result, it has become

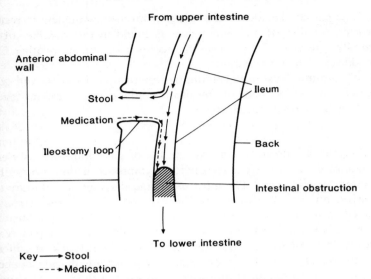

Figure 4 Diagram of a Bishop–Koop ileostomy.

possible for many infants with meconium ileus to have a much simpler operation. In the new operation the most obstructed part of the bowel is simply removed, and the two cut ends are joined.

It is a myth to suppose that children born with meconium ileus and thus diagnosed as having CF at birth are less prone to lung disease. While meconium ileus *almost* always implies the presence of CF in Caucasians, this is not invariable. Confirmation of CF by gene analysis or the sweat test is very important in any case of meconium ileus.

The most serious complication of meconium ileus is meconium peritonitis, an acute inflammation of the membrane that lines the abdomen (the peritoneum). Meconium peritonitis may be present at birth. It occurs when a hole develops in the wall of a section of bowel blocked by meconium. The meconium spills into the peritoneum and causes inflammation.

Attacks of incomplete intestinal obstruction may occasionally occur later in life from build-up of faeces and mucus. These have been labelled meconium ileus equivalent, but they bear no relationship to the condition affecting the newborn (see later in this section).

There is good evidence of a tendency for meconium ileus to recu
within families. If meconium ileus is found in one member of
family, there is a 50 per cent chance of it occurring in other C
children in the same family.

Meconium ileus or meconium peritonitis may affect the unbor
child and may occasionally result in spontaneous late miscarriage
stillbirth, or premature birth.

After the newborn period   Symptoms of gastrointestinal abnor
malities in CF are often seen before symptoms in the respirator
system or elsewhere. The most pronounced symptom is failure t
thrive, often with a ravenous appetite and oily or loose, strong
smelling stools, often associated with abdominal distension. Steatc
rrhoea is the indirect result of the fibrous scarring of the pancrea
from which CF derives its name. The fibrous tissue blocks the duct
of the pancreas and eventually stops the pancreatic digestive juice
from reaching the small intestine to digest the food, and in tur
causes nutrients to be inefficiently absorbed. Certain amino acid
do not depend on the pancreas for breakdown but are nevertheles
poorly absorbed, showing that the small intestine itself is no
functioning perfectly in CF.

Rectal prolapse   In this condition, malabsorption of fat, with ver
frequent stools, results in the inner lining of the rectum protrudin
through the anus. CF should be considered in any infant with
prolapsed rectum. Rectal prolapse should come under read
control if dietary fat is reduced and pancreatic enzymes are give
with the feeds.

Meconium ileus equivalent   This rather poor term is used fo
attacks of complete or partial intestinal obstruction that may occu
later on in the life of a person with CF. Attacks occur mainly as
result of blockage caused by mucus and fatty stools. In some Cl
adults abdominal pain and attacks of such obstruction may be th
main complaint. The condition is not more common among thos
who had meconium ileus at birth. Recent improvements in th
treatment of CF have reduced the incidence of this complication.

Intussusception In this disorder a portion of the small intestine folds into the adjoining region of the downstream bowel, threatening the blood supply of the trapped inner portion (see Figure 5). Intussusception is a rare but potentially serious complication of CF. Treatment is nearly always by surgery.

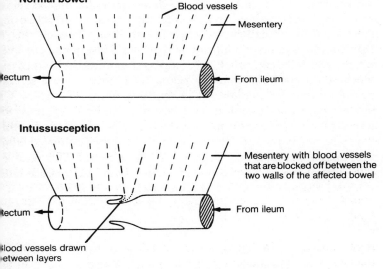

Figure 5 Diagram of intussusception.

Stricture of the large intestine Recently a number of children with CF have been described with fibrous stricture of the ascending colon of the large intestine. Children developed abdominal pain and vomited bile-stained fluid. This has been blamed on newer, stronger pancreatic enzyme preparations taken with the food (see p. 51).

The liver and biliary tree

Liver and biliary tree disease occurs in about 10–15 per cent of people with CF though it does not always progress to cirrhosis

(fibrous scarring) of the liver. In cirrhosis, the fibrous tissue lai
down partially blocks the veins draining into the liver from th
intestine and spleen. As the fibrous tissue contracts (part of th
natural progression of any fibrotic process), the liver cells may b
damaged. As a result they are unable to carry out their norma
tasks. The partial blockage of the blood supply to the spleen cause
it to enlarge, and the veins at the lower end of the oesophagus ma
also become swollen and varicosed. These varices (or dilated veins
may bleed on occasion and require the injection of sclerosin
agents, which strengthen the blood vessel wall. Though this i
a potentially serious complication that can cause jaundice, live
failure, and bleeding, in CF it is more common to see mild cases
which run a course over many years. Even after a more seriou
manifestation, the condition may improve. Why only a few Cl
patients have this complication is not fully understood. It is no
necessarily the older or the more severely ill who are affected in thi
way. The newborn with CF may sometimes show prolonged jaun
dice, possibly because of mucus in the bile channels. This resolve
with time and is not especially associated with liver disease late
in life. Gallstones are found in about 10% of CF adults.

Diabetes

Most children with diabetes have so-called insulin-dependen
diabetes. Two hormones, insulin and glucagon, are produced b
the pancreas, in groups of cells known as the Islets of Langerhans
Glucagon is produced by alpha cells in these regions, while insulir
is produced by beta cells. Insulin lowers the levels of sugar (glucose
in the blood by converting it to the carbohydrate glycogen, which i
stored in the liver. Glucagon is one of the hormones that reconvert
glycogen to glucose.

In insulin-dependent diabetes most of the beta cells (those manu
facturing insulin) are destroyed. However, diabetes in people with
CF is caused by contraction of fibrous scar tissue, which destroy
limited numbers of both alpha and beta cells. The resulting diabetes
which may first appear in the early teens, is generally mild and
easily controlled with small doses of insulin. The more severe com
plications of diabetes such as coma and acidosis (a build up of acids

in the blood) are unusual. Long-term kidney complications do not occur. About 3 per cent of adolescents and adults with CF develop diabetes.

Rare gastrointestinal manifestations in CF

Oedema is a generalized body swelling caused by low levels of the protein albumin in the blood. Albumin is involved in the process of keeping fluid in the blood vessels. When albumin is deficient, fluid builds up in the tissues. Oedema is sometimes found as a sign of cystic fibrosis in young infants. On occasion this has happened when the first loose stools have been misdiagnosed as milk allergy and soya feeds have been given.

Absence of gastrointestinal symptoms

A small proportion of people with CF have no problems with their digestive system. Some studies claim that as many as 10 per cent of CF patients show no gastrointestinal problems. The diagnosis of CF may be suspect in some of this 10 per cent. On the other hand, if one only suspects CF when there *are* gastrointestinal symptoms, one may underdiagnose this category of patients. There is undoubtedly a well-described group of pancreatic sufficient CF patients, in other words, people who have a pancreas that functions normally or close to normal. In fact the pancreas of these patients does show substantial tissue destruction but even a small (less than 5 per cent) amount of functional tissue is enough to produce adequate digestive enzymes. The majority of people with CF who have pancreatic sufficiency have genetic alterations that have a milder effect on the functioning of the CFTR gene product than does the $\Delta F508$ mutation.

The sweat gland

Sweat consists of a weak solution of electrolytes (electrically charged molecules) in water. These are mainly sodium and chloride, with some calcium and some potassium. The electrolyte solution has the same pH as the blood, being slightly alkaline. In CF there is a marked increase of these electrolytes in the sweat, because the re-absorption of chloride is impaired. It is known that the basic defect in CF is expressed as an abnormal regulation of the movements of salt across the layer of cells that line certain specialized ducts such as the sweat gland duct. Unlike other organs affected by CF, the sweat gland and its duct appear normal when examined under the microscope.

The reproductive system

One of the most consistent findings in men with CF is an abnor-mality of the epididymis and vas deferens (the tubes that carry sperm from the testes (see Figure 6)). These tubes end in blind channels instead of connecting through to the urethra. In fact, the epididymis is usually blocked and the vas deferens may be com-pletely absent. During fetal life, the male genital duct system ap-

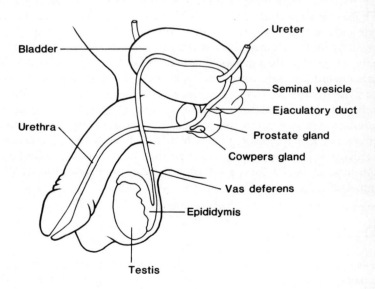

Figure 6 Diagram of the male reproductive system.

pears intact in CF. It seems likely that at some time before birth the duct system becomes blocked by mucus secretions as occurs in the pancreatic duct in CF. This blockage may then result in gradual destruction of the vas deferens. At least 97 per cent of males with CF are affected in this way from birth. As a result, most men with CF are sterile, although there have been documented cases of men with CF producing normal sperm and, in a few instances, of fathering children.

Of great interest is the discovery of certain rare CF gene alterations in sterile men with bilateral absence of the vas deferens and no other signs of CF. By some definitions these men could be said to have a very mild type of CF.

There are no equivalent changes in the female reproductive tract, and increasing numbers of women with CF are giving birth to children. Occasionally, reduced amounts of the mucus that normally lubricates the female reproductive tract cause infertility in women with CF.

How is a diagnosis of CF confirmed?

Sweat test

In most circumstances, CF can be confirmed in children by a carefully performed sweat test. In the sweat test, a small amount of pilocarpine (a sweating promoter) is driven into the skin by stimulation with a few amperes of electric current (this process is known as iontophoresis). When the sweating rate is adequate, the concentrations of sodium and chloride (i.e. salt) in the sweat are measured.

In a normal child the sweat will contain sodium and chloride in concentrations of between 15 and 30 millimoles per litre (mmol l^{-1}). Concentrations of sodium and chloride greater than 70 mmol l^{-1} are diagnostic of CF. This means that children with CF have two to five times the normal amount of salt in their sweat. A concentration of sodium and chloride well above 70 mmol l^{-1} does not indicate that the disease will be more severe.

The sweat test is quite safe and very reliable, but it needs to be performed by experienced staff. Stimulation of an adequate sweating rate in very young infants can sometimes be a problem. The

A brief summary of how CF may announce itself
at different ages

In the newborn:
   intestinal obstruction caused by meconium ileus or atresia;
   prolonged jaundice.
Infants:
   rectal prolapse;
   recurrent loose stools;
   distended abdomen;
   'milk allergy';
   recurrent chestiness, coughing, or wheezing;
   a salty taste to the sweat;
   poor weight gain, often associated with a ravenous appetite;
   unexplained dehydration.

   Because such symptoms are very common and may sometimes be
   mild, the diagnosis can be overlooked in infancy.

In older children:
   after the diagnosis of CF in a brother or sister;
   incomplete intestinal obstruction;
   nasal polyps, especially if recurrent;
   bronchiectasis or recurrent chest infections;
   heat prostration;
   underweight child.

   Occasionally the diagnosis may be missed for many years.

In adolescents or adults:
   delayed onset of puberty;
   sterile or azospermic males;
   infertile females with scanty cervical mucus;
   bronchiectasis.

recent introduction of a system that employs capillary pressure to
suck up sweat into polythene tubing has made sweat testing easier
and more efficient.

The sweat test is the least unpleasant method of diagnosis. In
cases where the results of this test are borderline, it may be necessary

o measure the pancreatic secretions directly, and check whether these secretions are reaching the duodenum. For this test it used to be necessary to insert a small tube into the duodenum via the mouth, but the test can now be done more simply by taking a urine sample and measuring substances in the urine that depend on pancreatic function.

It should be noted that in people with CF who have no intestinal troubles (see earlier section), the pancreatic secretion results would be near normal.

Occasionally, CF may go undiagnosed for many years, in which case the disease could be recognized in an adult. For adults, the normal range of salt concentration in sweat is greater than for children, and the sweat test rather loses its value in diagnosis. Men thought to have CF can be tested for azospermia (absence of sperm in the ejaculate). Since the discovery of the actual gene defect (see Chapter 7) a diagnosis of CF can now be made in about three-quarters of cases by DNA analysis.

DNA-based tests

Since the discovery of the actual gene defect, a diagnosis of CF can now readily be made in about three-quarters of cases by DNA analysis (see Chapter 7). This involves testing a DNA sample for up to a dozen relatively common errors in the CFTR gene that cause disease. However, since not all errors can be readily detected, as some are very rare, the sweat test still has a key role in diagnosis.

Other tests

In adults where CF is suspected for the first time, the sweat test rather loses its diagnostic usefulness. This is because high sweating rates may cause raised salt levels even in the absence of CF since the sweat gland is unable to reabsorb salt fast enough. In such cases a measurement of the electric charge across the cells that line the nose (nasal potential difference) can be useful. This test can only be carried out in specialist centres.

Should we screen the newborn for CF?

The validity of testing all newborn babies for CF is still a matter of debate. A simple test (BM Meconium) exists, which works on the principle that the albumin content of the meconium is increased in newborns with CF. This has been used in some countries over the past decade. A more reliable test is the measurement of serum immune-reactive trypsin (IRT) in a specimen of blood. This test is based on the observed reaction of the body's antibody defences to the pancreatic enzyme trypsin. A raised level of the antibody is found in the blood of most newborns with CF.

The problem with using the IRT test alone is that it has a relatively high false-positive rate. This means that of every 20 babies that are initially detected as having a raised IRT level, on average only one actually has CF. Hence, most of these 20 babies are quite healthy, but on occasion their parents are put under unfortunate and unnecessary stress when the possibility of CF has been raised. Using direct CF gene analysis in combination with the diagnosis of a raised IRT level makes the test much more precise. One in three babies that have a raised IRT *and* a positive gene test have CF. Of the others, some are healthy carriers.

Following the isolation of the CF gene it will soon be possible to detect CF by a simple test carried out on the genetic material of the majority of babies at birth. All that will be required will be a very small blood-sample, such as that currently taken routinely as a 'heel prick' from all new born babies to test for another inherited disorder called PKU (phenylketonuria). At present (spring 1994) such a test of the genetic material could only detect about 85 per cent of people with CF in the UK and possibly rather less than this in southern European populations. It is likely that before long nearly all CF individuals will be identifiable by this method.

Advantages and problems of screening

The most controversial question relating to newborn screening for CF is whether the eventual prognosis is altered by early diagnosis. This remains extraordinarily difficult to prove. Unfortunately, the strongest argument for screening remains the ease with which a diagnosis of CF may be overlooked, some children having had symptoms for a long time before the diagnosis of CF is considered or made. In one study, the *average* delay between onset of symptoms (excluding meconium ileus) and diagnosis was 13 months. This delay can cause psychological problems—parents may feel guilty about not noticing ill effects earlier, or may blame the general practitioner for not recognizing the symptoms when he first saw the child.

By allowing very early diagnosis, screening would sometimes prevent the birth of a second affected child.

When a truly effective early treatment for CF becomes available, capable of greatly reducing damage to the pancreas and lungs, then the case for screening will be made. Until then, it is important that paediatricians educate themselves, general practitioners, and the public about the early signs of CF.

4   Treatment of cystic fibrosis

The CF clinic—a multidisciplinary approach

Treatment of CF in a special clinic allows a local body of expertise to build up, to help manage the many complex ways in which the illness can affect a person. Greater longevity and improved health have been directly ascribed to special clinic treatment as opposed to care of the child by the paediatrician or medical practitioner alone.

An efficient CF clinic has a team of trained staff. The members of the team will vary from centre to centre. The team is led by a paediatrician and consists of a nurse, who works exclusively with CF patients (she has home and hospital contact with the families); a physiotherapist interested in lung function; a dietitian; a psychologist and/or a psychiatrist; and a social worker. The parents are the most important members of the treatment team, and later the child him/herself. Continuity is the greatest secret of success. The clinic at the Royal Manchester Children's Hospital (RMCH) is based on this model. Recently we have also had the services of a community physiotherapist who is able to visit children at home. An improvement in the children's and parents' understanding and performance in physiotherapy has been noticeable. We believe patients can be better treated at a special CF clinic than at a respiratory or gastrointestinal clinic that includes patients with CF.

Many children with CF live some way away from the CF centre. Shared care between the clinic and the local paediatrician is becoming popular. One American study showed that the long-term outlook for CF patients was closely related to the frequency with which they were seen by health professionals. Obviously, shared care increases the efficiency of disease surveillance.

With improved survival, more 'adult' CF clinics are coming into being. The age at which patients move to the adult clinic varies according to local facilities and expertise, but it may be as early as

16 years old. In some centres the physician and paediatrician run joint clinics and achieve continuity that way.

At the RMCH the 80 patients we have at present attend the weekly clinic by appointment where possible, though at any other time an open-door policy operates to clinic attendance and to the in-patients' ward. The patient and parents will see the paediatrician on each visit to the clinic, and often see other members of the team informally in the large anteroom containing the scales and lung-function equipment. Team members might check on aspects of dietary care, or the efficiency of the parents' physiotherapy techniques, in this way. Of course if a specific problem arises requiring detailed involvement of one of the team members (for example the psychologist), special arrangements can be made.

On a normal visit to the clinic, a patient is weighed, their height is recorded, and various measurements of lung function are taken. In addition they will see the physiotherapist. An instrument called a spirometer is used to measure lung function. The patient breathes

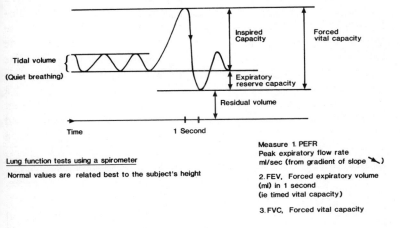

Figure 7 Diagram to show the theory of lung-function tests.

Key Forced vital capacity = total volume of air that can be moved
Inspired capacity = volume of air taken into the lungs on breathing in
Expiratory reserve capacity = the extra volume of air that can be breathed out
at the end of quiet expiration
Residual volume = the air which remains in the lung after deepest expiration

ROYAL MANCHESTER CHILDREN'S HOSPITAL
CYSTIC FIBROSIS OUTPATIENT CLINIC

Date:[   ]First Name:[   ] Surname:[   ]
Age:[   ]
General Comments:_____

_____

_____

_____

_____

Cough:[   ] 0.None 1.Occasional 2.Daily 3.Nocturnal 4.Exercise
Wheeze:[   ]   0.None 1.Occasional 2.Regular 3.Exercise
Exercise Intolerance:[   ]   0.None 1.Slight 2.Moderate 3.Severe 4.House Bound

Sputum Amount:[   ] 0.None 1.After Physio 2.Little 3.Moderate 4.Lots
Sputum Colour:[   ]   1.White 2.Yellow 3.Green
Haemoptysis:[   ] 0.None 1.Streaks 2.Moderate 3.Profuse

Chest Physio frequency per day:[   ] Forced expiration technique:Y/N
Who does physio:[   ]   1.Self 2.parents 3.Both 4.Other carer

School days missed per month since last visit:[   ]

Appetite:[   ]   0.Normal 1.Reduced 2.Increased
Stool frequency per day:[   ]   Smelly stools: y/n
Stool consistency:[   ]   0.Normal 1.Loose 2.Bulky 3.Hard

Constipation: y/n   Abdominal swelling: y/n
Abdominal pain:[   ]   0.None 1.Occasional 2.Moderate 3.Frequent
Pancreatic supplement:[   ] 1.Creon 25 2.Pancrease HL 3.Nutrizym 22 4.Other
Enzymes per meal:[   ] Enzymes per snack:[   ] Enzymes per day:[   ]

Hyperalimentation: y/n   Gastrostomy: y/n   Nasogastric feeding: y/n
Nutritional supplement: y/n Specify:

Immunisation:
Pertussis: y/n   Measles: y/n Hibs: y/n BCG: y/n Influenza: y/n
If no, please explain:

Drug Name	Route	Dose	Freq.	Duration
Flucloxacillin	O			long-term
Ketovite tab no:	O			long-term
Ketovite liquid(ml):	O			long-term
Vitamin E(mg):	O			long-term
Salt supplement(mmol)/day:	O			long-term

Kyphosis=round-shouldered stooping.
Troughing=sucking in of lower chest with breathing in.
Recession=sucking in between the ribs with breathing in.
Ausculation=listening to chest through a stethoscope.
FEV = Forced expiratory volume (see Fig. 7).
FVC = Forced vital capacity (see Fig. 7).
PEFR = Peak expiratory flow rate (see Fig. 7).
N–Crispin score = Crispin and Norman, a scoring system for
chest X-rays based on chest shape, lines, rings, shadows,
and opacities. The lower the score the better.
Anthropometric score compares the height versus weight centiles.

EXAMINATION:

Breath rate(/min):[   ]   Pulse rate:[   ]   Temp(°C):[   ]

Clubbing:[   ] *0.None 1.Nail bed hypertrophy 2.Watchglass 3.Drumstick*

Sternal bowing:[   ]   Kyphosis:[   ]   Troughing:[   ]   Recession:[   ]

0.Absent 1.Mild 2.Moderate 3.Severe

Wheeze:_____

Crackles:_____

Breath Sounds:[   ]   *0.Normal 1.Reduced*   Bronchial breathing: y/n

Heart Sounds:_____   Right ventricular heave: y/n

Ears:_____   Nose:_____   Pharynx:_____

Abdomen:_____

HEIGHT(CM):	FEV₁(L):	FVC(L):	PEFR(L/s):
WEIGHT(KG):	FEV₁(%):	FVC(%):	PEFR(%):
% WEIGHT FOR HEIGHT:	FEV₁/FVC:		

PUBERTAL STAGE (1-5)	BREASTS	PUBIC HAIR	PENIS	TESTIS VOL (ML)

Chest x-ray done today: Y/N

Date of last sputum test:_____

PS AERUGINOSA: Y/N	ROUGH: Y/N	STAPH AUREUS: Y/N	H INFLUENZAE: Y/N
	SMOOTH: Y/N	PS MALTOPHILIA: Y/N	ASPERGILLUS: Y/N
	MUCOID: Y/N	YEASTS: Y/N	OTHER:

PS CEPACIA: Y/N
Sputum/cough swab today: y/n

Other investigations:_____
_____
_____

Psychologist involvemnt:[   ]   *0.No   1.Previous   2.Current   3.Future*

Summary:_____
_____
_____
_____

Seen by:[   ] *1.Consultant   2.Registrar   3.SHO   4.Research Fellow*

Next appointments(weeks):[   ]

COMPLICATIONS		ITEMS	SCORE
NASAL POLYPS	Y/N	NORMAN-CRISPEN	
MECONIUM ILEUS EQUIVALANT	Y/N	LUNG SCORE	
CIRRHOSIS/ PORTAL HYPERTENSION	Y/N	ANTHROPOMETRIC	
SPLENOMEGALY	Y/N	GENERAL ACTIVITY	
COR PULMONALE	Y/N	SHWACHMAN-KULCZYCKI	
PNEUMOTHORAX	Y/N		
DIABETES MELLITUS	Y/N		
PANCREATITIS	Y/N		

JCC HUNG/ 1993

Figure 8 A CF clinic recording chart or proforma. (From the Royal Manchester Children's Hospital Cystic Fibrosis Clinic.)

into this apparatus, which measures the air capacity of the lungs, plus the speed and volume of air moved in and out of the lungs in breathing (see Figure 7). Also at each visit a cough swab or sputum sample is taken to check the current bacterial flora of the lung.

The findings of the physical examination are recorded on a proforma (figure 8), along with information on the patient's lung and bowel condition, their school or work attendance, and their treatment. The proforma is the one used at RMCH. We are encouraging neighbouring clinics in our region to use the same proforma so that computer comparisons can be made between patients at different clinics. We have recently introduced a summary sheet, updated approximately once a year. This contains important basic data needed for ready reference and which is also useful when patients are involved in research studies.

After each clinic session, a round-table discussion of those people seen at the clinic or in the ward takes place between all the staff members. Aspects of management and any planned or on-going research are discussed in practical terms at this meeting. Patients are seen a minimum of once every three months at the RMCH clinic, but many have more frequent contact through home visits from the CF nurse.

The hospital-based social worker has close contacts with many families and is especially involved with one-parent families and those with pressing financial or domestic problems. While she helps the families over various difficulties she has the opportunity of getting to know them well and to ensure that contacts with the clinic are maintained and attendance is regular. She acts on the families' behalf in processing claims for attendance allowance. From her training she complements the work of the clinical psychologist and clinic nurse.

The CF clinic: advantages and disadvantages

Advantages of a special CF clinic include improved health and life expectancy. A body of expert knowledge builds up and engenders confidence that the clinic is up to date with the latest advances in treatment. A camaraderie builds up between the children, their families, and staff members, and there are improved research opportunities. Contact with subjects with more advanced disease and knowing affected people who die may be numbered among the disadvantages.

A question relating to CF clinics that is frequently asked is, 'Can one "catch" a *Pseudomonas* infection from someone else attending the clinic?' One very good study in Dublin has shown that only brothers and sisters tend to share the same *Pseudomonas* species. *Pseudomonas* is a very widespread micro-organism in nature, being found in any drainpipe, for instance. Person-to-person spread of the organism is likely to be of minor importance in CF.

Recent new methods of typing *Pseudomonas* strains, using differences in their genetic material, shows that there is some cross-infection of *Pseudomonas aeruginosa* between patients, though this seems to be at a low level. In Copenhagen, Denmark, an attempt to keep people with *Pseudomonas* apart from those who were not yet colonized, resulted in a lower rate of infection. Recently at RMCH we have been alternating *Pseudomonas* and non-*Pseudomonas* clinic days. Cross-infection is much more likely to occur in confined spaces than in the open air and we have not changed our policy of taking children on camping holidays together, regardless of their *Pseudomonas* status, though we do arrange that bedrooms are not shared by those with *Pseudomonas* and those without.

A new finding in a number of CF clinics is the emergence of *Pseudomonas cepacia*. Called an epidemic strain, due to its infectious properties, not necessarily its virulence, *Pseudomonas cepacia* has been found to be considerably more infectious than *Pseudomonas aeruginosa*. Most instances of cross-infection have resulted from close social contacts in adults. Out-patient clinics are considered to be areas where the risk of cross-infection is low. We do, however, make sure that within our CF clinic we see our patients with *P. cepacia* after we have seen our patients who have *P. aeruginosa*. Unfortunately we have had to exclude our patients with *P. cepacia* from our CF holiday camp, though arrangements have been made for them to go on holiday together and with other groups of people with different diseases who are not at risk from *P. cepacia*.

One difference between *P. aeruginosa* and *P. cepacia* is that the former is widely present in the environment and the first acquisition

Table 1 Clinical evaluation and grading criteria for patients with cystic fibrosis

Points	Case histories	Lungs, physical findings, and cough	Growth and nutrition	Chest X-ray
25	Full activity Normal exercise tolerance and endurance Normal strength Normal personality and disposition Normal school attendance	No cough Normal pulse and respiration No evidence of over-expansion Lungs clear to stethoscope Good posture No clubbing	Maintains weight and height well within normal range, or just like the rest of the family Good muscle development Normal amount of fat Normal sexual maturation Good appetite Well formed, almost normal stools	Normal
20	Slight limitation of strenuous activity Tires at end of day or after prolonged exertion Less energetic Low normal range of strength Occasionally irritable or lethargic Good school attendance	Occasional hacking cough Clearing of throat Resting pulse and respiration normal Mild over-expansion Occasional, usually localized, harsh breath sounds, wheezing or rattling mucus heard Good posture Mild clubbing	Maintains weight and height at slightly below average or the family normal Good muscle development Slightly decreased fat Slightly retarded sexual maturation Normal appetite Stools more frequent and slightly abnormal	Signs of excess air in slightly over-distended lungs

15	May rest voluntarily Tires after exertion Moderately inactive Slight weakness Lacking spontaneity Lethargic or irritable Fair school attendance	Mild chronic nonrepetitive cough in the morning on arising, after exertion or occasionally crying, or occasionally during the day No night cough Respiration and pulse *slightly* rapid Barrel chest Coarse breath sounds Occasional localized mucus rattling or wheezing Moderate rounding of shoulders Moderate clubbing	Maintains weight and height at lower end of normal and less than other family members Weight usually deficient for height Fair muscle development Moderately reduced fat Abdomen slightly distended Maturation definitely retarded Fair appetite Stools usually abnormal, large floating, occasionally foul, but formed	Excess air in over-distended lungs Distance from front to back of chest increased Diaphragm pushed down Blood vessels in lungs prominent Patches of lung with less air than normal
10	Limited physical activity and exercise tolerance Breathless after exertion Moderate weakness Fussy, irritable, sluggish, or listless Poor school attendance, may require home tutor	Chronic cough, frequent, repetitive, productive, and rarely paroxysmal Respiration and pulse moderately raipd Moderate to severe over-expansion Widespread sounds of wheezing and mucus rattling	Weight and height below normal Weight deficient for height Poor muscle strength Marked reduction in fat Abdomen distended Failure of sexual maturation and no adolescent growth spurt	As above, but more marked Heart shadow narrow from pressure of lungs

Table 1 Clinical evaluation and grading criteria for patients with cystic fibrosis (*continued*)

Points	Case histories	Lungs, physical findings, and cough	Growth and nutrition	Chest X-ray
10 (ctd)		Rounded shoulders and forward head Marked clubbing Usually blueness of tongue	Poor appetite Stools poorly formed, bulky, fatty, and foul-smelling	
5	Severe limitations of activity Breathless when standing or lying down Inactive or confined to bed or chair Marked weakness Apathetic or irritable Cannot attend school	Severe paroxysmal, frequent, productive cough, often associated with vomiting or blood in sputum Night cough Rapid pulse or respiration Marked barrel chest Generalized squeaking, bubbly noises, and wheezing heard Poor posture Severe clubbing	Malnourished and stunted Weak, flabby, small muscles Absence of fat Large, flabby, protruberant abdomen Failure to grow or gain weight, often with weight loss Bulky, frequent, foul, fatty stools Frequent rectal prolapse	Marked overdistension Cystic spaces between areas of lung receiving too little air

This system of clinical evaluation can be used to evaluate patients at each visit or at six- or twelve-month intervals in order to determine the severity of the disease and the effect of therapy in any one patient and to compare one patient with the next.

The physical findings and chest X-ray are the best indicators of the degree of lung involvement and may be used without the other indicators to simplify and shorten the scoring. After Shwachman H. and Kukzycki L. T. (1958) Long term study of 105 patients with cystic fibrosis: studies made over a 5–14 year period. *Am. J. Dis. Child*, **96**, 6–15.

of the organism is *not* usually from contact with other infected patients. On the other hand the majority of cepacia infection does follow contact with other infected patients. This organism has interfered with the fellowship of patients with CF.

Specific aspects of CF management

Chest X-ray films are taken at least once a year. These are scored according to an accepted system to allow formal comparison. In addition, a Shwachman score is estimated yearly. This score gives points on the basis of well-being, school attendance, chest symptoms and signs, growth and nutrition, and the X-ray results (see Table 1). Both scoring systems allow a more objective approach than is allowed by simply reacting to findings at any particular clinic visit. At RMCH we also perform occasional chest scans on patients. These involve injecting and inhaling safe radioactive substances into the body. These penetrate the air and blood supply of the patient's lungs. Photographic scans of the chest may then show areas of the lungs receiving too little air or blood (see Figures 9a and b). Such areas may not be detectable by X-rays or with a stethoscope, and this makes the occasional performance of these other tests necessary.

The different tests of lung function are fairly variable and are more useful as indicators of long-term changes rather than being immediately useful.

Lung-function tests can, however, have immediate use in detecting a bronchospasm (contraction of the bronchial tubes). Sometimes bronchospasm may be suspected but cannot be detected with a stethoscope. In these circumstances, lung function tests are carried out before and after administration of a bronchodilator, a substance that relaxes the bronchial tubes. If bronchospasm is present, then the bronchodilator will improve the condition, and this will show on the second lung function tests. A bronchodilator drug can then be prescribed to ease the bronchospasm.

Immunization Immunization against those organisms that cause respiratory illness is essential in CF and should be available to children of any age. In particular, this applies to measles and pertussis (whooping cough), and unless there are very strong reasons not to, these inoculations should be performed. Annual immunization against the prevalent influenza strain is needed.

The manufacturers of the influenza vaccine advise its use above the age of four years. However, many paediatricians will recommend influenza immunization in younger children, too. Recently a vaccine against *Haemophilus influenzae* has become available (HIB). Its use for immunization of all children is being generally recommended and children with CF are no exception to this.

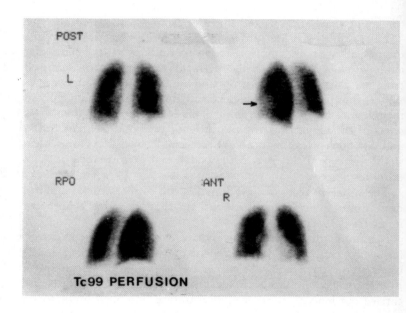

Figure 9 A lung scan. Different panels show the lungs from different angles.

Perfusion tests are on the blood supply to various parts of the lung. Black areas in the photographs are caused by radioactive emission, and denote lung tissue that is well perfused or ventilated. White areas denote areas where the radioactive isotopes have not penetrated, some of which are normal and simply indicate the positions of the heart and spine. Other white areas denote parts of the lung that are poorly perfused.

General aspects of CF treatment

People with CF are encouraged to lead as normal and as active a life as possible. Children with CF who swim regularly, for instance, show improvement in their lung function and well-being. A cough is no bar to sporting activity, although, obviously, breathlessness does limit the activity of some.

Despite ignorance of the basic defect in CF, multidisciplinary treatment has greatly prolonged life and its quality, so that reaching adulthood in reasonable health is becoming the rule rather than

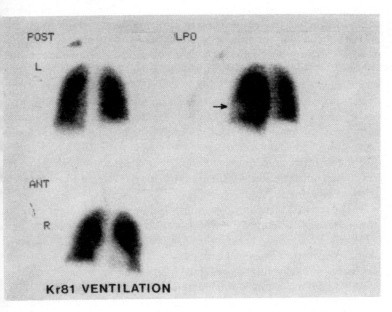

The two arrows in the figure mark an area of lung that is poorly perfused and ventilated. This area was not obvious on listening to breathing with a stethoscope or on routine X-ray. Once found, special physiotherapy was applied to this particular zone.

Key   Tc99 = technetium   radioactive isotopes that are inhaled (Tc99) or given
      Kr81 = krypton   by injection (Kr81)
      L = left   R = right   LPO = left posterior oblique
      POST = posterior   ANT = anterior   RPO = right posterior oblique

the exception. However, the severity of symptoms in individuals is highly variable, and very severely affected children may still die of the disease at a relatively young age, despite excellent treatment. More disturbing are patients who are initially only mildly affected but enter a more serious category simply through neglect of treatment.

Though there are many contributing factors, the improved survival in CF has been largely due to the development of effective antibiotics against *Staphylococcus* bacteria and to more effective treatment of *Pseudomonas* infections. Flucloxacillin and the more expensive fusidic acid are the most common antibiotics used to prevent and treat staphylococcal infections. There remain differences in practice between different clinics. Some, including ours at RMCH, believe in long-term (year-in, year-out) antistaphylococcal treatment, using full therapeutic doses of either antibiotic mentioned above, given by mouth. We are able to eradicate the staphylococcal infection from the majority of our patients in this way. Other clinics prefer to treat a staphylococcal infection vigorously if it occurs. We believe that this can only be done safely in a CF clinic with frequent testing for bacteria in sputum (phlegm) and careful surveillance. One danger of treating only when infection occurs is that the family might not want to bother the doctor with a 'trivial' infection and some lung tissue damage may occur as a result of the delay in treatment.

A theoretical argument against long-term treatment of the staphylococcal infection is an idea that these bacteria may help prevent a *Pseudomonas* infection. There is no evidence to support this idea. Another question often raised about long-term treatment is whether the continual use of antibiotics can make these drugs less effective. Unlike many other bacteria, there is at present no evidence for *Staphylococcus* developing 'immunity' to the effects of antibiotics in CF.

The very first *Pseudomonas* infection is often of the rough type. Early diagnosis of this infection in young children or in those not producing sputum may be made by a cough swab. Testing the blood for naturally circulating antibodies against *Pseudomonas* may also allow an early diagnosis of the first infection. A study in Denmark has shown some success in clearing the first infections with *Pseudomonas* by using a combination of two antibiotics, Ciprofloxacin® by mouth for two weeks and Colomycin® twice daily by inhalation, using a compressor and nebulizer for 3 months. Many clinics now follow this regime.

Pseudomonas infections may be difficult or impossible to eradicate. Once a mucoid *Pseudomonas* infection has become established it is generally a permanent feature, sometimes but not always resulting in worsened lung function.

It is generally agreed that patients with mucoid *Pseudomonas* need long-term treatment. This is given either by use of intermittent courses of intravenous antibiotics, by long-term inhaled antibiotic, or both, with occasional use of Ciprofloxacin® by mouth. Intravenous treatment used to be possible only with admission to hospital. However, trained CF nurses now enable many children and adults to complete their treatment at home, perhaps after a day or two in hospital for intensive physiotherapy and to allow medical and dietary assessment. Cannula design (the tube through which the antibiotics enter the blood stream) has improved so that many people on intravenous treatment can continue attending school or work. Most intravenous courses last about two weeks. The antibiotic chosen generally depends on tests of the *Pseudomonas* in the particular patient's sputum against a panel of antibiotics, choosing one (or sometimes a combination of two) to which the *Pseudomonas* is sensitive. The antibiotics used most commonly are one of the cephalosporins—Ceftazidime® or combination of a penicillin (such as azlocillin) with an aminoglycoside (such as Netilmycin®). Colomycin® or Tobramycin® are the drugs that are used most commonly by inhalation. Carefully controlled studies of patients on these treatment regimes have shown increased well-being and fewer days off school or work in people treated this way. Physiotherapy plays an important additional role, with the infection only suppressed by treatment and not eradicated. This is especially so in *Pseudomonas cepacia* treatment, since often this organism is unresponsive to any of the known antibiotics. *P. cepacia* often coexists with *P. aeruginosa* types in the sputum and appropriate antibiotic treatment may then be directed at the latter.

Difficulties of the treatment of pseudomonal infection are that most of the drugs used have to be given by injection, and the drugs may have unwelcome side-effects. However, it is rare to see the usual adverse effects on hearing and kidney function from these drugs in CF. Ciprofloxacin® is an effective anti-*Pseudomonas* agent that can be taken by mouth and is thus rather attractive. However, bacteria become resistant to it fairly quickly (though they may sometimes regain their sensitivity). Reports that Ciprofloxacin® may cause severe arthritis in childhood have been questioned recently. Though this may occur it is likely to be rare.

Some way of rendering the conditions in the lung less ideal for the *Pseudomonas* bacteria would seem the only way of eradicating pseudomonal infections. One approach has been to vaccinate against the bacteria, but this proved ineffective. A much more sophisticated *Pseudomonas aeruginosa* vaccine has been prepared recently. Unfortunately its use has been withheld due to fears that ridding the lung of *Pseudomonas aeruginosa* might make the patient more susceptible to infection by *Pseudomonas cepacia*. Whether this is really the case is currently being investigated.

Genetically engineered human DNAse (see Chapter 8) may help to suppress *Pseudomonas* infections by clearing the debris in which the organisms thrive.

Amiloride, a diuretic that blocks absorption of sodium ions, has been shown to correct partially the basic defect in the lung epithelium in CF. As a result this drug was given by inhalation in an American trial. Though bronchial mucus was found to become thinner after its use and the agent was found to have a weak anti-bacterial effect, no dramatic improvement in the health of amiloride-treated CF patients occurred.

Cough suppressants or stimulants do not help CF patients with chest problems. This is because such compounds relieve symptoms but allow mucus to remain in the lungs, thus impairing their function.

In some patients with CF, there is bronchospasm with wheezing. This may be associated with the CF or may be due to the very common chest condition, asthma. Bronchospasm in CF patients is treated in the same way as asthma. Inhalation of the drug cromoglycate may be used to prevent bronchospasm. On occasion bronchodilators (such as salbutamol) and steroids that act on the lung surface (such as beclamethasone) may be given to some patients by inhalation. Inhaled steroids, sometimes accompanied by oral steroids, may also be useful in controlling lung inflammation in CF.

Very occasionally, the airways may be washed out under anaesthetic (bronchial lavage) in an attempt to clear accumulated secretions preventing aeration of parts of the lung. In extreme cases a segment of lung with permanently dilated bronchi may be surgically removed. In some CF clinics in the USA and Canada such treatments are undertaken rather more often than in Great Britain.

Physiotherapy in CF

A fit person breathes more efficiently than an unfit one, especially when exercising. Someone with CF who is fit and has 'trained' their respiratory muscles is able to cope with the stresses of a chest infection more easily than an unfit person.

It is precisely when the child is well that physiotherapy and chest muscle training are important. Some children and parents seem to think that paying attention to physiotherapy when the child has a cough is sufficient. Mucus in CF is relatively dehydrated, but if there is infection and the bronchi are dilated, secretions of mucus and sputum can be very copious. Clearance of these secretions is paramount in allowing maximal ventilation of the lungs. Young children swallow their sputum, so the fact that none is being coughed out does not mean that no sputum is being produced.

In CF the upper lobes of the lungs are particularly prone to attack, although the reasons for this are unknown. The techniques employed in improving the strength and efficiency of the muscles of respiration and the clearing of sputum include breathing exercises (see p. 48), chest clapping with cupped hands, and sitting or lying in various positions to help mucus drainage (see Figure 10). The paediatrician may direct the attention of the physiotherapist and the parents to an area that requires special attention, because of physical signs found on examining the chest or on an X-ray or scan.

Physiotherapy

The aim of physiotherapy is to drain as much infected material from the lungs as possible and to ensure that there is no unnecessary build-up of thickened secretions in the airways. Techniques differ according to the age of the patient—in young children there is really no alternative to chest clapping and techniques of drainage where the child is placed in various positions to help drain different parts of the lung. As the child becomes older he or she can cooperate in more active self-help. The techniques of self physiotherapy which have proved to be most effective (as gauged by lung function tests and well-being) are active cycles of breathing exercises.

There are three components—

> breathing control
> chest expansion
> huffing or forced expiration technique.

The first of these is ordinary breathing at the patient's own normal rate and is interspersed between the other two techniques—its object is to avoid fatigue or increased bronchospasm which may sometimes interfere with the efficiency of physiotherapy. Chest expansion exercises consist of slow, deep inspiration as far as one can go, followed by ordinary relaxed expiration. Generally one would do three or four of these, followed by a period of breathing control, with or without chest clapping. Secretions are then further mobilized by the forced expiration technique—this consists of a huff, which narrows the small airways and forces mucus upwards; it is followed again by a period of normal breathing. These techniques are repeated in a cyclical fashion, usually for about 20 minutes—huffing is performed at various degrees of chest expansion—about halfway through quiet expiration, once or twice, followed by quiet breathing, then once at high lung volume after deep inspiration. It has been shown that such huffing is even better than coughing at mobilizing sputum. A parent or the patient can obtain quite a good idea about the amount of secretion in the bronchi needing clearing by the sound of the huff—a rough, rattly sound indicates uncleared secretions, as does any period of coughing; if the huff has no rattly quality and there is no cough, this indicates that secretions have lessened.

The period of normal breathing between the other manoeuvres can depend to an extent on chest symptoms (whether there is bronchospasm), and well-being at the time. It is widely accepted that regular physiotherapy is important, whether or not the person has chest symptoms at the time. During periods of well-being, twice-daily physiotherapy suffices, otherwise it may be increased to three or four times in a day. Chest clapping remains important, especially in younger children unable to use cyclical breathing techniques, and often forms part of the cycle during the deep inspiration mode in older children. Postural drainage also still has a role in helping to drain specific parts of the lung. Earlier editions of this book have included diagrams of positions for postural drainage of specific lung segments. Some positions are used far more than others and the photographs in Figure 10 (p. 48) show children in some of the commoner positions.

With accumulation of secretions from the previous night, morning physiotherapy is important. People who are able to play active sport or do swimming or exercise training could substitute this for one of their physio sessions as long as they still have at least one formal session a day. Sport should be encouraged in those with CF who are well enough, as it often improves psychological as well as physical well-being. Some children have a trampoline and bouncing on this can form part of a physio session.

If one suffers from bronchospasm, using a bronchodilator before the session or soon after the start is important and will result in far more efficient physiotherapy. Recently the drug DNAse (Dornase Alfa (Pulmozyme®)) has become available in various countries, including Britain. It appears to have a beneficial role in those people with moderate disease and chronic cough. It works by breaking down the DNA from bacterial and cellular debris in the bronchi. Thus it does not combat the basic defect in CF but, like many other therapies, helps to control the effects of the disease. Currently, doses and methods of administration, via a compressor with a nebulizer, largely follow the advice of the manufacturers. However, with more widespread availability of the drug and following research into more efficient methods of delivery into the airways, there are likely to be some changes in the way it is used. In particular, it may be possible to use lower doses of this expensive drug. At present it is not clear whether everyone would benefit from it but most doctors are likely to want to use it in their patients who produce sputum.

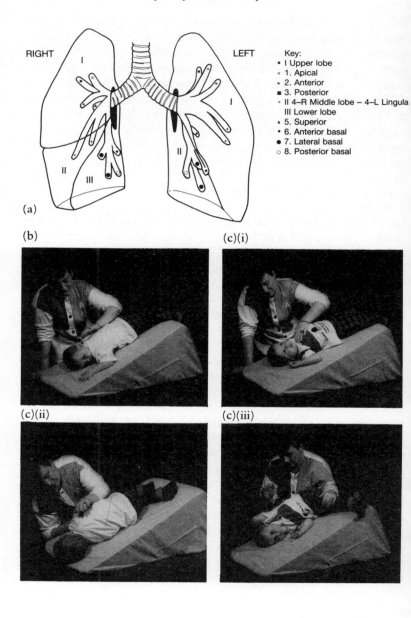

RIGHT   LEFT

Key:
■ I Upper lobe
× 1. Apical
◆ 2. Anterior
■ 3. Posterior
✛ II 4–R Middle lobe – 4–L Lingula
   III Lower lobe
▲ 5. Superior
● 6. Anterior basal
● 7. Lateral basal
○ 8. Posterior basal

(a)

(b)   (c)(i)

(c)(ii)   (c)(iii)

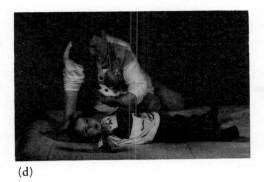

(d)

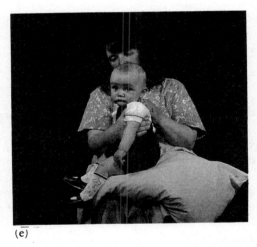

(e)

Figure 10 The best positions for postural (bronchial) drainage. (a) Diagram showing the names of the various lobes of the lung. (b) Posterior basal segments: the foot of the table or bed is raised about 50 cm (30°). Patient lies on abdomen, head down, with pillow under hip. Therapist claps over lower ribs close to spine on each side. (c)(i) Anterior basal segments: the foot of the table or bed is raised about 50 cm (30°). Patient lies on back, head down. (ii) Right lateral basal segments. (iii) Left lateral basal segments. (d) Anterior segments: lying flat. Therapist claps between collar bone and nipple on each side. (e) Apical segments: can be done sitting up or leaning back on a pillow at about a 30° angle. Therapist claps over the area between the collar bone and the top of the shoulder blade on each side.

Some centres use mechanical aids in physiotherapy, either on a routine basis or to help tide people over periods when they are too ill to perform physiotherapy. The positive expiratory pressure or PEP mask is popular in some centres—this keeps the alveoli and smaller airways expanded by causing expiration to start against a resistance. Although we do not yet know whether long-term use of this technique might aggravate emphysema, during times of airway instability the technique may be helpful in improving lung function and well-being. Nasal continuous positive airway pressure or CPAP has been used to reduce the work of breathing in people with advanced disease who are becoming exhausted by the effort of normal breathing. One of its uses has been to keep patients on the active transplant list alive, while a donor is awaited.

Nebulized antibiotics are given after the physiotherapy session, to give the antibiotic the chance to stay in the respiratory tree until the next physiotherapy session.

Nutritional and dietary aspects

Dietary needs in CF are increased to about 130 per cent of normal. This results from a combination of the effects of the cellular defect in the disease, increased loss of nutrients in the stool, and the effects of chronic lung infection. In the days before the introduction of acid-resistant enteric-coated pancreatic microtablets or granules, it was difficult to give sufficient pancreatic enzymes with meals to cover the increased dietary requirement.

The introduction of enteric-coated microtablets or granules, resistant to the effect of stomach acid and thus released for the first time in the duodenum and small intestine, where naturally pro-duced pancreatic enzymes would enter the bowel, has resulted in far better absorption of dietary fat and protein. The unpleasant effects of malabsorption (the production of frequent, foul-smelling stools) are now rare. However, large amounts of the enzymes, Pancrease®, Creon®, or Nutrizym® may be needed to achieve adequate absorption of food. The dose of enzymes needed to allow normal growth and normal stools differs from patient to patient.

This is because of differences in the absorptive surface of the small intestine and varying transit times taken by food to pass through the gut. Enzymes should ideally be given throughout the meal and not simply at the beginning or end. In young babies or children, granules from opened capsules should be given in something slightly acidic, like apple sauce. If the granules are placed in milk, for instance, the enteric coating protection will be lost and unprotected enzyme destroyed by stomach acid. Children who complain of abdominal pain and loose stools may be forgetting to take their enzymes, especially with snacks. Because of the large numbers of capsules needed—sometimes as many as 20 with a meal—there was pressure to introduce a capsule with increased lipase. High lipase capsules were introduced in 1992 and did allow a reduction in capsule numbers, though not as great as one might have predicted from these triple-strength preparations (Pancrease HL®, Creon 22®, Nutrizym 25®, and Panzytrat®). Unfortunately, use of these preparations has resulted in a new complication in a number of children—narrowing and stricture of the ascending colon of the large intestine, (see section on complications of treatment, p. 00). However, some patients have felt so much improved on these high-lipase capsules that they and their paediatricians have decided to continue using them.

As lung disease becomes more advanced there may be increased difficulty in taking in sufficient calories in a normal diet. High-energy milk shakes, like Fortisip® and Fresubin® and calorie additives like Polycal® can prove useful, especially as snacks before bedtime or at times calculated not to interfere with appetite at main meal times. Sometimes poor appetite or a persisting inability to gain weight require a more active approach to treatment.

Night feeding of high calorie and energy protein–fat hydrolysates given during sleep by drip, using a fine polythene tube passed via the nose, gullet, and thence into the stomach have helped many to gain weight. Many of those people with CF who have used this way of feeding are very pleased with it and there are children of primary-school age who have learned to pass their own tubes. The treatment is not recommended for those with recurrent night coughing, since in these circumstances the tube could become coughed out of position with the danger of food entering the lungs.

Even more efficient night feeding may be achieved by gastrostomy, a minor operation in which a soft, fairly large-bore tube is inserted into the stomach through the left side of the abdomen. This route may be used over a period of many months or even years, although the tube needs to be replaced from time to time.

The newer technique of 'button gastrostomy' is associated with many fewer side-effects than is conventional gastrostomy. The technique involves a smaller incision and a cosmetically neater appearance but has the same advantages of excellent weight gain and increased well-being. Gastrostomy is quite often recommended for patients accepted onto heart–lung transplant waiting lists, as improved nutrition improves the chances of a successful operation. Occasionally parenteral nutrition (feeding of high-energy solutions by vein) has been used in the same way. There is quite good evidence of an improvement in lung function in patients whose nutrition has been improved by any of these methods.

Occasional patients persist with steatorrhoea despite huge doses of pancreatic enzymes. In some of these patients an elegant group of drugs that reduce the amount of acid produced by the stomach and aid its emptying, may result in improved absorption of food in the gut. (Examples of these drugs are cimetidine and ranitidine.) Although such drugs are effective in treating people with peptic ulcers, it does not seem desirable in CF to interfere with the normal working of the stomach over long periods of time, so their use is limited to special situations.

Salt

There are increased salt needs in CF, particularly in hot weather. Certain children seem particularly prone to acute salt depletion and the need for extra salt should be considered in any child with CF who shows signs of lethargy. Occasionally, during a heatwave, a child may become weak or dehydrated and may need a saline solution to be given intravenously. Dietary salt is often cited as a cause of high blood pressure, but in CF this is not the case, because increased salt in the sweat provides a safety mechanism.

Vitamins

Supplements of the fat-soluble vitamins A, D, E, and K are needed because of the malabsorption of fat. Night blindness and dry skin have been described in patients with CF not taking vitamin A. Similarly, bruising and bleeding from vitamin K deficiency has been described, as has poor balance that is associated with vitamin E deficiency. These complications do not occur in people who take the appropriate vitamin supplements. Though vitamin D levels are low in CF, rickets has never been described. Ketovite® tablets (three per day) and Ketovite liquid (5 ml per day) supply adequate amounts of vitamins A, D, and K. Vitamin E tablets (Efynal®) satisfy the vitamin E needs and are recommended for all CF patients.

Trace elements

Some elements, such as iron, selenium, and zinc are found in very small amounts in the body. They are necessary for certain body functions (for example, iron is an integral part of haemoglobin, the molecule that transports oxygen around the blood), and must therefore be taken in the diet. Low levels of zinc and selenium have been found in people with CF but treatment with these substances has not led to any noticeable benefit.

Treatment of other symptoms of CF

Meconium ileus equivalent

An increased dosage of pancreatic enzymes is the first approach to treating this condition. Surgical treatment of meconium ileus equivalent may occasionally be necessary, but most attacks can be managed by increasing liquid intake and by administering water-attracting enemas (such as Gastrographin®) or drugs like acetyl cysteine (which thins the intestinal mucus). (Attempts to use the mucus-thinning properties of acetyl cysteine to treat lung complications in CF have proved fruitless, as the action of the drug was found to be too vigorous.) Lactulose is also frequently used in the further prevention of repeated episodes of meconium ileus equivalent.

Rectal prolapse in infancy comes under control once the steatorrhoea is treated. Children with strictures associated with high lipase pancreatic extracts have needed surgery, sometimes with half of the colon being removed.

Diabetes

As mentioned earlier, the diabetes in CF is generally mild and small doses of insulin suffice to control it. There are generally some modifications needed in the diet, and a diabetic with CF would need to ensure that salt intake was adequate. We at RMCH generally share the care of diabetic CF patients with a diabetes specialist.

Nasal polyps

Some people with CF develop outgrowths of the mucous membrane inside the nose, nasal polyps. These are about the size of a small pea, on average, and may cause moderate inconvenience by blocking the nostrils. Sometimes numerous polyps are removed by surgery. Unfortunately, recurrence is quite common. Local cortisone (steroid) preparations sniffed into the nose may cause polyps to shrink in size, rendering surgical removal unnecessary.

Liver disease

Milder and earlier involvement of the liver is detected more frequently, especially in centres which routinely perform annual blood tests of liver function or ultrasound examination of the liver. There is general agreement that oral administration of ursodeoxycholic acid (known as URSO) helps bile acids and salts to pass through the liver into the bile, reducing the build-up in liver tissue which may result in cirrhosis, and improving liver function.

It was explained in Chapter 3 (p. 22) how varices or dilated veins occur at the lower end of the gullet in people with cirrhosis of the liver. People with varices must avoid taking aspirin or similar ubstances, as these drugs may cause bleeding. Individuals with varices may need to take vitamin K and drugs of the cimetidine group to reduce stomach acid. Occasionally, sclerosing agents may be needed. These drugs strengthen the walls of the blood vessels, thus making bleeding less likely. These are injected directly into the varices, under anaesthetic.

Complications of treatment in CF

Antibiotics

Any drug may, on occasion, produce side-effects. Most of the treatment given to patients with CF is remarkably free of side-effects. To some extent this may be because as part of the basic defect of CF, the kidney clears certain drugs out of the body at an abnormally rapid rate. This allows large doses of a drug to be given without the usual complications. A good example is the aminoglycoside group of drugs like gentamycin or tobramycin which may affect the inner ear and cause deafness. Despite generous doses this is very rare in CF patients.

Ciprofloxacin® has the capacity to cause joint pain, sometimes severe. Because of anxieties that it may affect growing cartilage, the manufacturers recommend its use only in adults. As it is an effective oral agent against *Pseudomonas aeruginosa* there has been a strong temptation to use it in children. Parents counselled about what has turned out to be a very small risk of joint pain in childhood allowed the drug to be used. There have been recent publications stressing the safety of Ciprofloxacin® in children. Ciprofloxacin® forms part of the standard treatment when *Pseudomonas* is isolated from a cough swab or sputum for the first time.

Pancreatic enzyme supplements

A large number of enteric-coated pancreatic capsules may need to be taken with meals to allow an adequate caloric intake to be digested. There was pressure from patients and doctors on manufacturers to introduce more concentrated capsules with a higher

lipase content. Keen competition between the three main manu
facturing firms resulted in each company introducing a high-lipase
product more or less simultaneously in 1992. For Creon 25®
Pancrease-HL, and Nutrizym 22, it was thought that doses could
be cut by one third because of their higher concentration. Most
patients changed over to the high-lipase preparations with relative
ease, though for most the new dose was closer to one-half than one
third. Many found the change very convenient, and some gained
weight better than previously. The majority maintained their nutri
tional state on the new capsules, showing no other benefit than the
considerable added convenience of fewer capsules. Unfortunately i
appears that these higher strength capsules are not as safe as lower
dose ones: at the end of 1993 in England nine boys were described
who had developed a stricture in the ascending colon of the large
intestine after taking the higher strength preparations for about
18 months each. An operation was needed to remove the stricture
and surrounding abnormal bowel. In some patients hemicolectomy
or removal of half the colon, has been necessary to allow bowel
contents to be passed freely again. These children had had no other
change in their management other than the altered pancreatic for-
mulation. The complication was described with all three brand
and with a fourth, less used in the UK, Panzytrat®. Recent views
are that a dose of 15 000 units of lipase per kilogram body weight
should be the maximum dose per meal, with a total daily dose not
exceeding 40 000 units per kilogram.

The Committee on Safety of Medicines contacted all doctors at
CF clinics and thereafter all doctors in Britain, recommending a
return to lower dose preparations. Some specialist centres who had
never encountered the complication, despite using very large doses
of the high lipase preparations, have decided to keep patients on
these. In most other centres the stronger capsules have only been
retained in children whose clinical condition had improved greatly
on them and whose nutritional state had been causing concern on
the weaker strength capsules. Early evidence is that the majority of
children have changed back to the weaker preparations without
difficulty. Some have reported improvement in their digestion, as
if the stronger capsules with lower numbers of granules in the
intestine had been less effective.

Fertility and CF

Adults with CF often ask for counselling about fertility. Nearly all men with CF are sterile and their ejaculate contains no sperm. Nevertheless, in a small percentage of cases this is not so, and men with CF have been known to father children. In addition, in some cases, functional sperm may be collected directly from the genital ducts upstream of the blockage. Women with CF are fertile, though they may have abnormal cervical mucus and may sometimes come to infertility clinics. Some women are not well enough to be able to undertake pregnancies, but an increasing number of women with CF are having children.

Pregnancy

Sadly, the cost of pregnancy is great for women with CF. Heart failure may occur, and lung function often deteriorates. In the only good study of its kind, 18 of 100 women who undertook pregnancies died within two years of giving birth, with 12 of them dying within six months. The chances of the baby dying within a few days of birth and of being premature were also increased in this group. Other factors that deserve consideration are the impact of the mother's shorter lifespan on her child and her possible inability to see to the child's daily needs. It is generally agreed that unless the disease is very mild, women with CF are best advised to avoid pregnancy.

Contraception

Oral contraceptives should be used with great care by women with CF, as they can cause blood clots in the veins. Oral contraceptives should be particularly avoided when there is liver damage (as in cirrhosis). For many women with CF, spermicidal jelly in conjunction with condoms is the method of choice.

The foregoing are many of the general aspects that might be dealt with when genetic counselling in CF is given. Specific details of tests of prenatal diagnosis are discussed in Chapter 7.

5 Heart–lung transplants and cystic fibrosis

A great deal of publicity has been given to the combined heart–lung transplant as a means of increasing the lifespan of children and the growing number of young adults with CF. Obviously this operation is only going to be available to a relatively small percentage of CF patients. There are still only a small number of centres in the UK with the expertise and facilities to carry out this major feat of surgery. Since these centres are also carrying out operations on all other relevant medical cases, the CF patients must take their turn on a long waiting list. People are not always suitable for heart–lung transplantation on medical or psychological grounds. Even when an individual has entered the transplant programme, having fulfilled all the necessary criteria, it may be a very long wait before he or she can be transplanted. Initially they are put on a provisional waiting list, where regrettably many patients die prior to having the opportunity of a transplant. The major delay, of course, is the shortage of donor organs. When a donor is identified it is then really down to the luck of the draw as to who on the waiting list has the same blood group (hence reducing the chances of rejection of the transplanted organs) and organs of about the same size of the donor.

If two potential recipients are equally well matched to a donor, then a clinical decision as to which of the two is sicker, and hence more in need of the transplant, will be made.

It must also be said that not all heart–lung transplant patients survive the operation nor the immediate problems of infection and organ rejection. Furthermore, we still do not know by how long this operation is capable of prolonging the life of a CF patient. Since the operation is a relatively new one, only time will answer the question. In other words, in the absence of effective treatment for the terminally ill CF patients who have entered the stage of lung

ailure, it is reasonable to attempt this relatively high-risk opera-
ion. However, it is hoped that in the longer term, as the major
advances in our understanding of CF that will follow on from the
solation of the CF gene (see p. 80) are transmitted into effective
reatment for lung disease, this operation may be superseded.

Clive Sandercock and Gary Gifford are two of the CF patients
who have received combined heart–lung transplants and more than
9 months after their operations they spoke to one of the authors
A.H.) about it.

Gary is now 23; he was diagnosed as having CF at the age of
18 months. As a child he was often sick, and was in and out of
hospital frequently until the age of 12 or 13. From then until he was
around 18 things went rather better, but the next two years saw a
relatively rapid deterioration in his health, and by the time he was
21 he was more or less unable to do anything that expended energy.
He had actually been an in-patient at the Brompton Hospital in
London for more than three months, relying on a continued oxygen
supply to survive before he received his transplant.

Clive is 30, has a relatively mild form of CF with no digestive
system involvement. An infection caught on holiday at the age of
14 turned into a severe chest infection which led to the diagnosis of
CF being made. Even though from this age onwards he always had
a cough and was frequently short of breath, it never seriously
impeded his life and his job as a mechanic. However, from the age
of 25 or 26 his health deteriorated quite rapidly. He was in the
Brompton Hospital for seven weeks before having the transplant.
Clive has a much rarer blood group than Gary and fortuitously a
matched donor became available relatively soon. Though more
potential donors with Gary's blood group became available, there
were obviously more patients with the same type on the waiting list
above him.

Both Clive and Gary described the wait for the operation, once
they knew they had been placed on the list, as by far the worst part
of the whole procedure.

Before the operation you know that every day you are going to get a little
bit worse and after it you are going to get a little bit better. Even very soon
after the operation you could start doing things that you wouldn't have

thought of doing beforehand, little things that to most people would seem like nothing but to yourself are big steps forward. For example, brushing your teeth. Before the transplant you just didn't have enough puff to do this, you would do three brushstrokes and then stop because you had run out of energy. Now, you just brush your teeth without thinking about it

Another difficult time was actually coming up to the Brompton Hospital, otherwise known as the National Heart and Lung Hospital, in the centre of London. Clive said that this was really quite a shock and he felt rather lost, too far away from home surroundings (both Clive and Gary come from the Cornwall and Devon areas) and that until he came to accept this move it was pretty tough going. To add to the problems at this stage, Clive was feeling really ill and his condition deteriorated over the next few weeks in the Brompton. He had so little energy that he was unable even to walk around his bed. Not only did lack of oxygen make him look blue but it also made him behave in slightly crazy ways, doing things which he later regretted, but which he was often not aware of doing at the time—for example, pulling out his catheters, and being aggressive to the nursing staff and doctors. Behaviour like this is certainly not in his nature!

Until the last few weeks before his operation Gary had tried to go outside for a short walk each day. He set himself something to look forward to every day and a challenge to meet, however small, even if it was only to walk up the hospital corridor. During his last few weeks at the Brompton he could not leave his hospital room, and he knew he never would without a transplant (he was on a continual oxygen supply and had no energy to move). He recalls that some days he felt so terribly ill that he could have given up and died, but that he made himself fight on.

The heart–lung transplant operations were performed at Harefield Hospital in Middlesex. Both Clive and Gary described the move to Harefield Hospital as 'great'. They were both warned that although a suitable organ donor had become available, it was at that stage far from certain that the operation would go ahead. Despite this, the overwhelming feeling was one of relief that at last the wait was over and that now they were going to have a chance of a successful operation. As Clive said: 'As long as I got to Harefield's and they did something then at least I had had my chance and it was my own fight after that.'

The actual heart–lung transplant operation obviously does not feature prominently in their memory of the whole story. Both had seen a video describing what was going to happen to them. When they actually first registered all that was going on around them (remarkably soon) after the surgery, they were surprised by how few external signs there were of what had just happened to them. The intricate machinery of monitors, catheters, blood bottles, and so on that are part of such a major operation were all hidden, either behind the bed-head or under the bed. All they could see were a few pacer wires attached to their body, and they did not even have a long line of stitches in their chest, the incision having been closed by laser 'stitching'. Of course, although their parents had been warned what they would see from the other end of the bed, they were still pretty shocked.

Clive remarked that though it was uncomfortable and they both felt rather 'beaten up and sore' after the surgery, they never actually felt any major pain associated with it. In fact, their arms and shoulders were very sore from the actual physical trauma they had suffered during the long operation. Their major worry at this stage was not disturbing their new set of organs by moving too violently or breaking open their wound during physiotherapy. It took Clive and Gary quite a long time to get fit again after the heart–lung transplant, mainly because they had been so ill for a long period before the operation. Their muscles were already wasted, they were very thin, and even lying in bed made them sore. Both spent five weeks in Harefield Hospital after the operation, and then several weeks in a flat in Harefield village which allowed them to be fully independent but yet to have the safety net of the hospital nearby, particularly during the early stages when rejection of the new organs can first become a major problem.

Gary describes his life after the heart–lung transplant as 'brilliant'! 'I've never had it so good, I'm doing all sorts of things that I haven't been able to do for years and never thought I would be able to do again.' He plays table tennis and five-a-side football. They are both so happy to be able to lead a relatively normal life again: to be able to get up in the morning, get dressed, and start their day rather than spending hours 'getting ready', doing physiotherapy, and so on; to be able to run down the road to get the morning paper rather than planning their trip to the paper shop around where and how often they could stop for a rest; to have the ability to take the stairs rather than having to use the adjacent escalator. They feel that their social lives are better because they have so much more self confidence.

Clive and Gary both admit that things have not been completely straightforward since their operation and that maybe they sometimes paint too rosy a picture. They do still get days when they don't feel well, but even when this happened soon after the transplant they could see that every day they were able to achieve something they could not do before. For the first few weeks they had a great deal of nausea and Gary suffered from fluid build-up, which put pressure on his lungs and liver. They were very apprehensive about the symptoms and side-effects of the operation, worrying that they might be signs of organ rejection. They suffered some depression, particularly when they felt they were not recovering as fast as some other heart–lung transplant patients had. An early worry also was whether or not the new pair of lungs was going to start deteriorating in function, as their own pair had done. They were encouraged to cough and clear their lungs, just as if they were doing characteristic physiotherapy for CF treatment. However, it now seems that, at least so far, their transplanted lungs are not showing any CF-related disease.

Several months later, they see the only major side-effects of their treatment as the continual need for immunosuppressant drugs (to prevent organ rejection) and the effects of steroids. The most noticeable feature of steroid intake is the marked effect it has in promoting the growth of hair, both on the face and the body. Obviously, though the young men do not mind this, it can be quite upsetting for young women.

When asked to summarize the most important attributes for a CF patient who is going to enter the heart–lung transplant programme, Clive and Gary homed in on the same points. First, they need a really positive attitude to life, and second, they need a solid family back-up. As Clive said, 'When you feel rough you have to think I've got to keep going, I've got to hang in there and wait; you must never think "I'd rather be dead". You need a lot of parental support and support from your friends to keep going.' In fact, both were sure they would not have got through the whole thing without parental support, and that it was actually more difficult for their parents than it was for them. Their parents felt so helpless, watching their sons going downhill fast, and then unable to contribute during the operation and recovery period, while at least Clive and Gary could contribute in a 'mind over matter' sense. Neither feels that opting for the chance of an operation that is so obviously risky and traumatic as a heart–lung transplant was a courageous decision. They felt so ill before the operation and knew that they were going to die, so that given any chance to feel better and prolong their life, they had to take it. As Gary said, 'I've always enjoyed life, even when I was feeling bad, and I so much wanted to live I just had to go for the operation.'

6 Psychology of cystic fibrosis

Many aspects of the disease CF, its chronic nature, uncertainties about long-term prognosis, the genetic aspects, and the impact on family life, to name but a few, can affect the psychological functioning of the affected person, individual family members, and the family as a whole.

The experienced CF clinic team can play an important role in recognizing early signs of psychological difficulties and in providing support and advice. Often the paediatrician may call on the expertise of the team's clinical psychologist.

People with CF, and their families, tend to be realistic about their situation and to cope with day-to-day and long-term problems. It does need to be emphasized that the illness itself and its treatment does impose a lifelong discipline on the individual and the family.

Cystic fibrosis affects people with widely differing temperaments and from diverse backgrounds. The reactions of various family members tend to depend more on these factors than on the CF condition itself. This said, there are specific occasions in the evolution of the CF when stress factors may be increased.

At the time of diagnosis

Since most diagnoses are made in early infancy or childhood, it is the parents who first experience psychological distress. The anxiety and frustration at the months of frequent visits to the doctor with complaints about their child's abnormal stools or recurrent cough may surface when the diagnosis is finally made. The relief that a diagnosis has finally been made is often tempered by the stark realization of what the diagnosis may imply. In earlier times, couples tended never to have heard of CF until the doctor presented them with the diagnosis in their child. Mass media (magazines, TV, radio) attention to CF will often mean that individuals have heard f the disorder, and often about some dramatic (newsworthy) aspect. Thus alarm at the diagnosis may be their first reaction.

Occasionally the diagnosis may have been missed for years. Then frustration and anger may be especially keenly felt, aggravated by fear of a worsened prognosis because of the delay.

Rejection of the accuracy of the diagnosis by the parents is seldom a problem where diagnostic tests were performed after the child became ill. However, diagnoses which follow on screening tests and with the child still healthy can understandably be challenged by parents, though the onset of symptoms is seldom long delayed.

The CF team is careful not to overwhelm parents with too much knowledge about the condition too quickly, and is available to provide a great deal of support in the early days. Frequent clinic and home visits enable parents to develop confidence about CF, its treatment and the long-term outlook.

Meconium ileus

Here there has been no delay in making the diagnosis. However, a dramatic operation within a few days of the child's birth, with the baby sometimes in an intensive care unit far away from home, causes its own stresses.

We know of couples who have been left with the abiding feeling that they could cope with a second child affected by CF but not with a second operation in the newborn period for meconium ileus. The nurse from the CF team is increasingly called by the intensive care surgical team to make the first contacts with the parents, to instil confidence about the future.

Childhood

Most young children with CF need to spend very little time in hospital, and require a minimum of injections. With better nutrition and improved pancreatic enzymes most will not stand out from their peers. However, for those who are more severely affected there may be problems with being underweight, with the recurrent severe cough, and with time off school. For some, with early *Pseudomonas* infection, there is the pain and discomfort of hospital admission and of the intravenous needles needed for antibiotic administration. Some children may be embarrassed by the number of pancreatic enzyme capsules they need to take with their school meals. Children have been known to discard or conceal their capsules. Some young children may rebel against their enforced inactivity during physiotherapy sessions, and elicit anxiety in their mother or father. Visits to the CF clinic may be times of stress for the parents, worried that some sign of deterioration may be found or that their fears in this regard may be confirmed. On the other hand, there is usually the reassurance that the check-up, discussion of problems, and adjustments in treatment brings, so parents and child often go home relieved that the situation is under control. Failure to keep appointments at the CF clinic is always treated seriously by the team, and may sometimes signify a psychological problem. Friendships between families develop at clinic or through CF organizations. News travels fast between some of the families about dramatic events, such as someone dying of CF or a heart–lung transplant that has occurred. Such events can explain temporarily increased levels of anxiety.

Adolescence

Adolescents with CF are no different from other adolescents in terms of concerns about the future, their looks, relationships with the opposite sex, etc. It is also a period of emerging independence when peer groups can be important. Parents rightly worry when an adolescent becomes rebellious and rejects treatment. Some adolescents may ask pertinent questions about their disease and begin to be more forceful in their views about treatment. This may involve requests for more home versus hospital intravenous antibiotic courses. They may express concerns about long-term survival, and the boys about sterility. Some adolescents may lag far behind their peers in terms of height and weight—this is especially, though not only, in the presence of advanced lung disease. People in this group may be prepared to undergo the inconvenience of nightly naso-gastric or gastrostomy feeding to increase the amount of energy taken in. Being underweight and undersized may dominate their thoughts.

Adulthood

There is a great camaraderie among many adults through the Associations for CF Adults. These articulate groups have vocalized some of the concerns and needs of affected adults and have helped many professionals understand their problems. Having a job is as important to the dignity and self-esteem of a person with CF as it is to any other person in our society. One dilemma which adults may face is whether to mention their disease to employers. According to the Association for Cystic Fibrosis Adults, 50 per cent of affected adults in Britain are employed, 18 per cent unemployed, and 3.6 per cent unable to work through illness. Of the remainder, about half are students and half housewives.

Reactions of individual adults to their illness differ widely. Some few regard the CF as a treasured part of their personality, while most regard the CF as a challenge, trying not to let the disease dominate their lives.

Relatively few men with CF marry (10 per cent), while 33 per cent of women do. People of both sexes with CF do form long-standing relationships. Perhaps the implications of being sterile may be a reason for the low marriage rate in males.

Affected women who decide not to have children need to consider sterilization as a preferred mode of contraception. Couples who decide that they do want children have to consider this option very carefully for a number of reasons, including the possible effects on the woman's health. An affected man and his wife may wish to have a child, using donor sperm. It would be important to ensure that the donor is not a CF carrier.

The Adult Association accepts the issue of prenatal diagnosis and termination of a pregnancy with CF as a matter of personal conscience. Understandably, this is a sensitive area.

The impact of new treatments

Most dramatic of these has been heart–lung transplant. The great majority of parents and of affected children or adults are positive about wishing to accept the offer when it is made. A prelude to this is the conversation with the doctor about the hopeless long-term prognosis without surgery. This conversation, however difficult, used to be the one to help the parents and child to prepare for the child's death. Now the offer of curative treatment may dominate this phase, and there needs to be counselling, generally undertaken by the transplant team, about the fine details of the procedure and preparation for it. For some there is the happy outcome of a successful transplant, for others death comes with the person still on a waiting list and sometimes with inadequate preparation. The CF team needs to exercise its medical and psychological skills to the full in helping the affected person and the family to cope with any outcome.

There is the comfort that everything possible was tried, which may help the parents to get over their grief, if the person does die. Not all those who have transplants survive, and it is difficult for the parents and CF team to remember that an 80 per cent survival chance includes a 20 per cent chance of failure. One additional source of pride to individuals and families may be the so-called domino procedure, where the heart of the CF sufferer is used in heart transplant while he or she receives a heart–lung transplant from another donor. The various difficulties still attendant on transplant are seen as an inevitable price for true progress.

Preparation for dying

Not all families are able to talk openly about the impending death, and sometimes parents or siblings are overwhelmed by grief. In other families there is quite open discussion between affected older children or adults and the family, and they have been able to bid farewell to family, friends, and members of the CF team. When death seems inevitable, a decision by the patient and/or parents is required as to whether it would be better for this to occur at home or in hospital. When home is chosen, a key worker from the CF team, often the CF nurse, will act as the main link between the affected person, the family, and the hospital. The aid of the general practitioner will generally be sought, and with the CF nurse arrangements are made for the dying person to be kept as comfortable as possible, with sedation where necessary. Some parents and relatives have found bereavement support groups helpful, others have found most comfort through their religion. The clinical psychologist can provide bereavement counselling where appropriate.

The parents and siblings

Cystic fibrosis may impose extra strains on the marriage, though some couples are drawn closer by it. The divorce rate is not higher among parents of a CF child than in the general population.

Healthy siblings may experience a number of difficulties. They may feel that they receive disproportionately less of their parents' time and thus feel neglected and resentful, with guilt feelings about their feelings of resentment. As they grow up, they may worry about their chances of being a carrier and their risk of having affected offspring themselves.

Mothers often carry the main burden of responsibility for treatment, with its taxing, daily demands. Of all the family members, including the affected person, mothers have been shown to have the greatest amount of knowledge about CF. They are also the most likely to become depressed from time to time. The depression is usually not so severe that they are unable to attend to all the demands of treatment. Rather, it manifests as 'feeling blue' or being tired. If the mother herself is ill the family may need a great deal of support.

Fathers, on the whole, involve themselves in the health and welfare of the child and in carrying out some of the treatment, especially physiotherapy. Where the father is the major wage-earner, this may limit his involvement and he may seldom be able to attend the CF clinic with his child. It may become habit for the father to opt out of assisting in the care of the affected child. Having an ill child may limit the family's earning capacity—it is difficult for both the mother and father to work, and choice of work or mobility are limited by the medical needs of the child. In countries where there is no national health service, the financial burdens of caring for a child or children with CF may be crippling.

Genetic aspects

The recent genetic discoveries have been hailed as great break-throughs. Nevertheless, affected people have been heard to say that, thus far, no affected person's illness has been helped as a result of these discoveries. Prenatal diagnosis and termination of pregnancy pose a dilemma, especially for a condition affecting one's beloved child and for which treatment, no matter how burden-some, is available. On the other hand, couples may not wish to 'inflict' the condition on another child and may fear being left childless, should the affected child die; and there is their wish to have a healthy child. When a decision is made after careful thought and counselling to opt for prenatal testing, there may be heightened anxiety associated with the chorionic villus biopsy, waiting for the results, and the one in four who are told that the fetus is affected and who have to decide on whether to continue with the pregnancy or to have a termination. The couples' experiences during earlier prenatal tests and whether they resulted in termination may affect their decision. Couples who have had a termination do not get over the experience easily, though there is some evidence suggesting that the earlier in pregnancy a termination occurs, the less the long-term psychological effects.

Religious convictions may help some couples in their decisions, while others may feel pressured by their religion.

The genetic counselling team provides the parents with full support, whatever they decide to do. This is likely to minimize any possible psychological difficulties arising from the responsible decisions of informed couples.

Professional help

When psychological problems are prominent, there is generally one member of the CF team to whom the patient or parents best relate and through whom any modifications can be suggested. By virtue of his or her training, the clinical psychologist is best equipped to deal with particularly difficult or entrenched problems. Sometimes, the psychologist will decide to work through one of the other team members, when that seems best for the patient or family.

Conclusions

All the psychological problems which may occur in CF are functions of the particular circumstances that surround that family. None are really specific to CF. These problems may change, as new treatments with different demands are introduced.

7 Genetics of cystic fibrosis

Introduction: mitosis and meiosis

The human body is made up of a huge number of individual functional units called cells. These cells are too small to be seen by the naked eye, but they can be looked at through a microscope in which they are magnified maybe fifty to one hundred times. Each cell is surrounded by an outer membrane, within which are a number of structures essential to the working of the cell. The nucleus is one of these. It is surrounded by another membrane, and contains among other things the genetic information of the cell. All the cells of an individual have the same genetic information. It is this information that is responsible for the inherited characteristics of an individual.

Body cells are continually dividing during life; in this way the body can grow and repair itself. When a cell divides, it produces two daughter cells, each of which contains the same genetic information as the parent cell. To achieve this, the parental cell genetic information is duplicated before cell division so that there are two sets of this information, one for each daughter cell. This type of cell division is known as *mitosis*.

When the cell is not dividing, the genetic material is spread throughout the nucleus. However, when the cell is about to divide, the genetic material contracts and coils up. As a result of these changes, the structures in each cell that contain the genetic material (known as *chromosomes*) can be seen much more clearly as specific structural bodies (see Figure 11). Chromosomes are asymmetrical structures consisting of a short (p) arm and a long (q) arm separated by a central constriction, the *centromere*.

Different species have different numbers of chromosomes. Humans normally have 46 chromosomes in all the cells of their body apart from the sex cells (the eggs or the sperm). Each of these body cells is *diploid*, i.e. it carries two complete sets of genetic information. Thus the 46 chromosomes consist of two sets of 23.

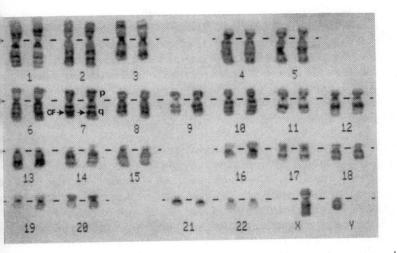

Figure 11 The chromosomes of a normal human male. The banding pattern, produced using a special stain, is characteristic of each pair of chromosomes. The CF gene is located half-way down the long (q) arm of chromosome 7.

One chromosome set comes from the mother via the ovum (egg) and the other comes from the father via the particular sperm that fertilized the ovum. Both ovum and sperm are *haploid*, that is they carry only a single set of 23 chromosomes. When egg and sperm fuse in fertilization, the chromosome complement of the ensuing embryo is restored to 46 (23 pairs).

In 22 of these 23 pairs of chromosomes, members of the pair are the same in men and women. These pairs are known as the *autosomes*. The twenty-third pair comprises the sex chromosomes, X and Y. Women have two X chromosomes, men have one X chromosome and one Y. Unlike the autosome pairs, the X and Y chromosomes are functionally dissimilar. The Y chromosome is very small in comparison with the X and apparently carries very little genetic information, apart from that required to direct male sexual development.

As has already been mentioned, the ovum and the sperm only carry a single set of chromosomes. Eggs and sperm are made by a

process called *meiosis*: a diploid cell with 46 chromosomes divide
into haploid cells containing 23 chromosomes each.

If meiosis simply involved one chromosome from each pair going
into each haploid cell, then the maternal and paternal chromosomes would remain unchanged from generation to generation and
there would be little genetic diversity. What actually happens is
that during meiosis the two sets of genetic information in the cell
are shuffled like two packs of cards. This process is known as
recombination.

Before the cell divides in meiosis, the chromosomes join in homologous pairs. This means that chromosome 1 inherited from the
mother joins up with the corresponding paternal chromosome, and
likewise chromosome 2, 3, 4, etc. pair up. Random and reciprocal
exchanges of genetic material then occur within each homologous
pair, involving sections of genetic material from one chromosome

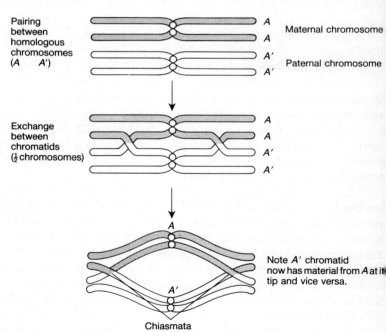

Figure 12 Diagram to show recombination at meiosis.

breaking off and replacing the equivalent section on the other chromosome (see Figure 12).

The two main chemical components of chromosomes are deoxyribonucleic acid (DNA) and proteins. It is the DNA that in its structure contains all the information needed to construct a human being from a single fertilized egg. The building blocks of DNA are chemical units of a base (a nitrogen-containing compound, either a purine or a pyrimidine) and a sugar molecule (deoxyribose) joined together. Many of these units are linked through phosphate molecules into a long chain (see Figure 13a). The four different bases that are used in DNA are called adenine (A), guanine (G), cytosine (C), and thymine (T). These are the elements of the genetic code (the 'language' of the genetic information). The DNA in chromosomes is in the form of a double chain, the so-called 'double helix', in which the two chains are wound round each other and joined together by their base units (see Figure 13b). The structure can be likened to a spiral staircase where the two continuous sides (sugar–phosphate back bones) are joined at regular intervals by the stairs (bases) (see Figure 13c). Due to differences in the sizes of the individual base molecules (adenine and guanine are bigger than cytosine and thymine), adenine can only join to thymine and guanine can only join to cytosine if the two sides of the staircase are to remain a constant distance apart.

Each DNA molecule can replicate itself, making an identical copy of its genetic information. This is what happens before mitosis, the cell-division process described earlier. However, for this genetic information to be useful to the cell, it must be translated into a form that can be used by the cell machinery outside the nucleus. To achieve this the DNA has to be copied, or transcribed into another molecule, ribonucleic acid (RNA), otherwise known as messenger RNA. In turn, this messenger RNA is used as a blueprint for the translation of the genetic message into biologically useful molecules, proteins. Proteins are made up of a long chain of building blocks, called amino acids, that are joined together to form a functional whole. The base sequence in the RNA copy of the DNA directs the insertion of a particular amino acid in a specific place in each protein. Each amino acid corresponds to a set of three bases occurring in the RNA, and the nature of these three base

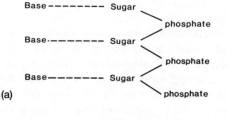

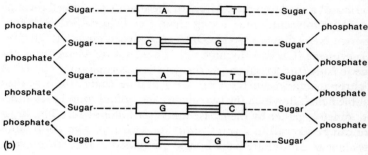

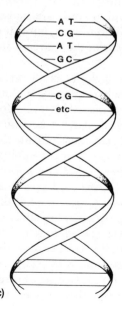

Figure 13 The structure of DNA. (a) The basic DNA chain. (b) Two DNA chains joined in a functional unit. (c) The double helix in three dimensions.

coding units and the particular amino acids they correspond to, is called the genetic code. For example, a run of three adjacent bases CTT in the DNA would result in insertion of an amino acid called phenylalanine at that point in the particular protein chain being made. Many thousands of different proteins are made in the one cell. Proteins can really be regarded as the primary product of genetic information and all the different proteins made in an individual are responsible for his or her uniqueness. They have a wide range of functions in the body: structural proteins are major components of muscle, skin, hair, and many other tissues, while enzymes are essential parts of the body's metabolic machinery.

Since all the cells in the body arise from mitotic division of the fertilized egg, each cell carries a full complement of genetic information, i.e. 46 chromosomes. However, only a very small part of this information is being used in any one cell at any one time. In fact, much of the DNA in the chromosomes never seems to be used at all in coding for proteins. The important coding regions of the DNA are found within functional units called *genes*. It is the coding regions within the genes that are transcribed into messenger RNA which then goes on to be the blueprint for protein manufacture, as we described above. Within and between genes or groups of genes are large non-coding regions of DNA. Some of these non-coding regions may have some role in controlling the activities of the genes, but the vast majority, as far as we know, seem to have no function at all.

The cells of a particular tissue or organ will have a specific set of genes in action. Hence, though the enzyme-secreting cells of the pancreas and the cells lining the respiratory system will have certain active genes in common, (that is those making products that are essential for the maintenance of any living cell), other active genes will be coding for products involved in tissue-specific functions. For example, the pancreas secretory cells will have active genes producing specific digestive enzymes to break down food, while genes coding for mucus will be switched on in many of the cells lining the respiratory tract.

It should be remembered here that each cell contains a pair of each gene, one from each parent. Genes coding for the same product can vary slightly in their precise DNA sequence from one person to the next. Where an individual has inherited identical forms (*alleles*) of a particular gene from both parents he is said to be *homozygous* for that gene, but if he has inherited non-identical alleles for any specific gene he is defined as *heterozygous* for that gene. The words *heterozygote* and *carrier* of a particular gene are in some cases interchangeable.

Genetic diseases are caused by abnormal genes that do not fulfil their proper function. An abnormal gene can be classed as dominant or recessive. If an abnormal gene is dominant, its abnormality is manifest even if the other gene of the pair is normal. However, when an abnormal gene is recessive, the abnormality is masked if the other gene of the pair is normal. So a person who has CF or a similar recessive hereditary disease must be homozygous for the

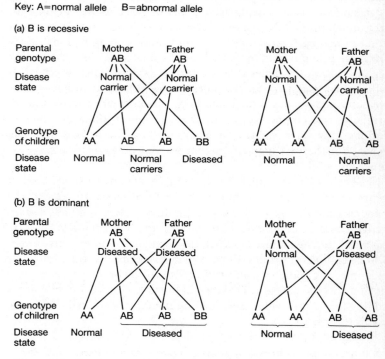

Figure 14 Diagram to illustrate dominant and recessive inheritance.

abnormal gene, i.e. they must have inherited the abnormal gene from both parents. An individual who is heterozygous (i.e. has one normal and one abnormal gene) for a recessive hereditary disease is known as a *carrier* of the abnormal gene. Carriers do not have the symptoms of the disease, but may pass it on to their offspring.

The combination of all the different genes that an individual has are known as his or her genotype. Simple inheritance patterns of dominant and recessive genes are illustrated in Figure 14.

Both dominant and recessive diseases can be subdivided into autosomal and sex-linked conditions, which are coded for by genes located on the autosomes or on the sex chromosomes, respectively. The known inheritance pattern of the CF gene, derived from the study of many affected families, shows that equal numbers of male and female CF children are born to healthy parents. From this pattern it is clear that the CF gene must be autosomal and not sex-linked. Recessive diseases coded for by a gene on the X chromosome, such as haemophilia, are much more common in males than in females. This is because a male has only one X chromosome and so there is no possibility of a normal gene masking the defective one. For a female to be affected she would have to carry the same defect on both of her X chromosomes, necessarily a rare event.

Cystic fibrosis is an autosomal recessive disease, i.e. affected individuals inherit a defective gene from both parents. We have known since 1985 that the CF gene is located on the long (q) arm of

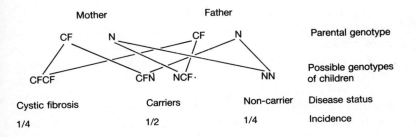

Figure 15 Inheritance of the CF gene from two carrier parents.
Key CF = CF gene   N = normal gene

chromosome 7 (see Figure 11). However, there is no visible abnormality in chromosome structure; the fault is a much more subtle change within the DNA molecule. The classical inheritance pattern of the CF gene from two carrier parents is shown in Figure 15.

The cystic fibrosis gene

The isolation of the cystic fibrosis (CF) gene in 1989 by the groups of Lap-Chee Tsui in Toronto, Canada, and Francis Collins in Michigan, USA was the culmination of more than five years' work by various research groups to move from linked DNA markers to the gene itself. Isolation of the gene opened a new and exciting chapter in CF research. It was now possible to start asking and answering fundamental questions about the molecular basis of the disease.

The structure of the CFTR gene

The gene responsible for the disease cystic fibrosis is called the cystic fibrosis transmembrane conductance regulator, CFTR for short. The protein that is coded for by the CFTR gene is called the CFTR protein. It was given this name by the researchers who identified it because they thought it regulates the movement of electrically charged chloride (salt) ions across the membrane surrounding specific cells in the body. The CFTR protein normally works to move salt out of these cells but in CF a defective protein is made due to errors in the CFTR gene and so normal chloride movement cannot take place.

In terms of human genes in general, the CFTR gene is large, spanning about 230 000 units of genetic information on the long arm of chromosome 7. In fact only a small part of this genetic information, 6200 units, actually codes for the message that directs the making of the CFTR protein. The coding region of the CFTR gene is made up of 27 individual units that are copied from the DNA of the gene and joined to each other in a chain (messenger RNA, see p. 75). The coding region directs the assembly of a protein containing 1480 amino acids, called the CFTR protein.

What does the CFTR protein do?

The CFTR protein probably looks something like the illustration in Figure 16. It appears to be anchored within the membrane surrounding the cells in which it is found and to form a pore in that membrane through which electrically charged chloride ions can pass out of the cell. The pore in the cell membrane is normally closed but when chloride needs to move out of the cell the CFTR protein changes shape to allow the pore to open. Figure 16 shows the important parts of the CFTR protein that protrude from the cell membrane into the cytoplasm of the cell. These are the two NBF* domains and the R* globe (explained at the bottom of page 82). The change in shape that accompanies salt movement is caused by other molecules within the cell binding on to the R segment and the two NBF segments of the protein.

Though it is clear that the movement of chloride through the pore in the cell membrane is one function of the CFTR protein, many researchers believe that the protein may have an additional function. This is partly because it is hard to see how all the features

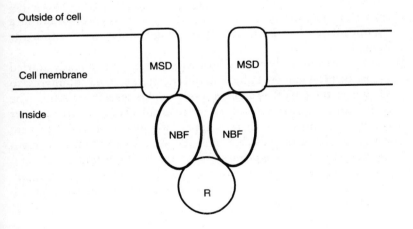

Figure 16 Important parts of the CFTR protein.

Key   MSD = membrane-spanning domain   NBF = nucleotide binding fold
        R = regulatory domain

of CF disease could be caused simply by a failure to move chloride ions out of some cells in the body. In addition, certain features of the structure of the CFTR protein suggest that it may also perform another function in the cell.

Where is the CFTR protein found?

As with many other important proteins that carry out highly specialized functions, CFTR protein is not found in all cell types and organs in the body. Expression of the CFTR gene in readily detectable amounts appears to be restricted to the layer of cells (called epithelial cells) that line certain organs. The majority of these cell layers are within the ducts of the organs, for example the pancreatic ducts, the sweat gland ducts, and the male genital ducts. CFTR protein is also found in parts of the layer of cells that lines the small and large intestine. This pattern of expression of the CFTR protein is perhaps to be expected, since, with the exception of the kidney, these are all tissues that are affected by the CF disease process. Surprisingly, given the central role of the lung in CF, there is very little expression of the CFTR protein in the layer of cells that lines the airways and the lungs. CFTR protein is only found at a significant level in particular types of glandular cells within the lung.

Since we know that the CF disease process has already started before birth, while the baby is still in the uterus, it was of interest to see where the CFTR protein is found in the developing fetus. The main surprise was that before birth (from about 12 weeks after conception until term) there is apparently plenty of CFTR protein within the layer of cells that lines the airways and lungs. At birth the CFTR protein disappears. This may be important in CF lung disease, but we do not yet understand how. There remain many gaps, such as this, in our understanding of how exactly the CF disease process happens.

---

* NBF actually derives its name from nucleotide binding-fold since the molecules that bind to these folds are called nucleotides. R is short for regulatory since the molecules that regulate the opening of the CFTR pore bind to this region.

Errors (mutations) in the CFTR gene

Over the past four years a large number of laboratories across the world have been identifying the disease-associated mutations in the CFTR genes of their CF patient population and contributing their data to the Cystic Fibrosis Genetic Analysis Consortium. This data collection has been coordinated by Dr Lap-Chee Tsui in Toronto for dissemination, on a confidential basis, to other contributing laboratories. The consortium has not only provided a pool of information and resources for participating laboratories, but also generated useful data on the population genetics of cystic fibrosis. Clearly, each research laboratory individually does not have sufficient numbers of DNA samples under analysis to generate useful population information. However, through the pooling of results several important aspects of the genetics of cystic fibrosis can be analysed. Two key questions are being addressed as a result of this. First, whether specific populations across the world carry specific mutations at a higher frequency than elsewhere. Second, whether it is possible to predict the severity of disease on the basis of the particular mutations that a person carries.

What types of errors in the CFTR gene cause cystic fibrosis?

The errors in the CFTR gene that cause CF are called mutations. These can occur in a number of ways that are summarized in Figure 17.

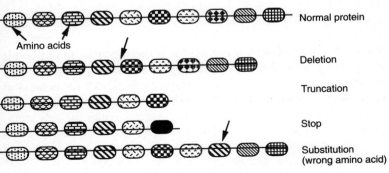

Figure 17 How mutations alter proteins.

Deletions

The most common mutation in Britain, North America, and most of northern Europe is the deletion of three coding units of DNA (CTT) resulting in the loss of one amino acid, phenylalanine, at position 508 of the protein (ΔF508). The effect of this mutation on the protein is to prevent the normal process of passage of the protein to the membrane of the cell (see Figure 18). CFTR protein builds up within the cell instead, where it cannot perform its usual functions. There are now many examples of other deletion mutations in the CFTR gene that have a variety of effects depending on their size and location within the gene. However, most of them result in the loss of one or two coding units so the wrong amino acids are inserted into the protein at that point and hence further along the protein too. The net result of this is usually a non-functional, truncated, or non-existent CFTR protein.

Stops

Another type of mutation which occurs relatively frequently in some populations is the change of a single coding unit within the DNA so that the mechanism of reading the sets of three coding units is signalled to 'stop' rather than to put the next amino acid into the protein. The effect of this is to make a truncated protein rather than full-length CFTR. These short, part-proteins are usually completely unstable and non-functional, if they are made at all.

Substitutions

A frequent type of mutation in CFTR is the substitution of a single coding unit in the DNA, changing the three-code unit and resulting in one wrong amino acid being inserted into the CFTR protein at that point. Many of the CFTR proteins with one wrong amino acid have been studied within cells. They usually reach the cell membrane and are correctly inserted into it, but then do not function correctly. Different amino acids have a wide range of biochemical properties that can greatly influence the three-dimensional structure and the activity of the whole CFTR protein.

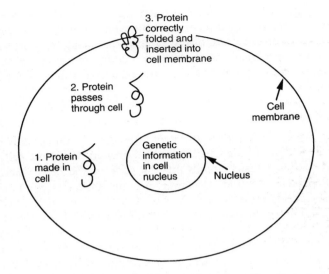

Figure 18 How CFTR protein is made and processed.

A particularly interesting group of substitution mutations comprises those that alter specific amino acids in the transmembrane portions of CFTR (see Figure 18) and that interfere slightly with the normal passage of chloride across the cell membrane. These mutations have been found in some CF patients with milder disease, including a normal pancreatic function, even when the other CF gene is the 'severe' delta F508. (Remember that mutations in *both* one's CF genes must be present before disease will manifest itself—having only one CF mutation results in being a carrier for the disease.)

Missassembly

The mechanism whereby the 6200 coding units of the CFTR gene are extracted from 230 000 total units in the gene is complex. Essentially, 27 segments of various lengths of coding units that make up the 6200 are extracted from a RNA copy (see page 75) of the whole CFTR gene and joined to each other. There are very precise signals built into the DNA units of the gene at the beginning and end of each of these 27 segments that cause the segments to become correctly joined together. Mutations in these signal regions can result in one or more of the 27 segments being left out, so that the message produced for the protein-making machinery is shorter than 6200 coding units. This usually means that normal CFTR is not made.

Regulation

At the moment we understand very little about what actually regulates the activity of the CFTR gene and protein within the cell. Nor do we know what 'switches on' the gene in the cells where the CFTR protein is found. However, it is likely that as our hunt for disease-causing mutations in the CFTR gene moves out of the 6200 unit coding region, we will start finding parts of the DNA that control the gene. By drawing parallels with other genetic diseases, we expect to discover that some mutations occurring in these control regions cause the CFTR protein not to be produced at all in some CF patients. The complete lack of the important CFTR protein within the specialized cells that normally express it then causes disease.

Questions

1. Do different mutations affect the severity of CF disease? This question is quite difficult to answer since it requires comparison of

Occasionally, when giving information to a CF patient about the particular mutations that they carry, a genetic counsellor may use what appears to be a code. This code is in fact quite simple and works as follows. Every amino acid in the CFTR protein has a number that denotes its position in the protein chain. In addition there is a single-letter code to denote precisely the type (chemical structure) of the amino acid. When an error in the gene causes the wrong amino acid to be inserted into the protein chain at that point, this is described by a letter–number–letter shorthand. For example, quite a common mutation in the CFTR gene is called G551D, which means simply that at position 551 in the protein chain the normal glycine (code G) amino acid has been replaced by an aspartic acid (code D) amino acid.

In the same code, the letter X is read as a 'stop' signal by the machinery that joins together the amino acids in the protein. The common mutation G542X means that at position 542 the normal glycine (code G) amino acid has been replaced by a signal to stop adding amino acids to the protein chain. The terms *ins* and *del* simply denote the insertion of extra unwanted coding units or the deletion of essential coding units in the CFTR gene. So *ins*1154TC means the insertion of a T and a C unit after the normal base 1154 in the CFTR message.

the disease process in a relatively large number of patients with each mutation. Otherwise, we could not be sure whether features of the disease were due to CF gene defects or to the effects of natural variation between individuals caused by other genetic and non-genetic factors. Even identical twins with the same mutations may not have the same severity of disease. Since most of the mutations causing CF (with the exception of ΔF508) are relatively rare, members of the Cystic Fibrosis Genetic Analysis Consortium have pooled their clinical data on patients with specific combinations of mutations so that they can compare the effect of individual mutations on disease severity. The only obvious trend to come out of this comparison is that CF patients who carry two ΔF508 CFTR genes are more likely to be pancreatic insufficient (that is to require enzyme supplements to help them digest their food) than are patients with a variety of other CF-associated mutations.

Mutations that cause 'stop' signals in the protein, as described above, were initially thought to result in less severe disease than the ΔF508 mutation. However, now that a larger number of patients and 'stop' mutations have been examined it turns out that the severity of disease may be highly variable and different 'stop' mutations may have different effects. Severity of lung disease and liver disease have not yet been shown to be closely associated with any particular mutations. Further, within each group of patients carrying the same mutations, even siblings, there is a remarkable range of severities of disease. In short, with the exception of severity of pancreatic disease it is not possible to predict the disease course simply from knowledge of the mutation within the CFTR gene. There are a very few alterations or mutations of the CF gene which do generally appear to cause milder, though still significant, disease.

2. Does the inheritance of different mutations from each of the parents affect severity?

There is no good evidence for the inheritance of different mutations from each parent having a direct effect on disease severity. Here again it has been difficult to collect data on a sufficient number of individuals with the same combination of two rarer mutations to rule out the effects of natural variation between individuals that has got nothing to do with the particular mutation in the CF gene. However, it would be generally true to

say that there is as yet no substantial evidence for different combinations of mutations affecting disease severity. It remains possible
that certain mutations that have relatively little effect on the CFTR
protein might partially compensate for a mutation having a pro-
found effect on the protein in the other CFTR gene of a CF patient.

3. Do different mutations require different treatments? The
answer to this question is no. Clearly patients with sufficient
pancreatic function not to require enzyme supplements are spared
this part of treatment. However, such patients (usually not carrying
the ΔF508 mutation in both their CFTR genes) are rare and often
progress to being pancreatic insufficient and hence requiring enzyme supplements as the disease proceeds. All other aspects of the
treatment for CF will rather be tailored to treat the current clinical
problems of the disease in an individual regardless of the mutations
that he or she carries.

**4. Do different mutations affect the outlook for future treatments
by drugs or gene therapy?** Current approaches to developing new
treatments for CF are largely aimed at 'bypassing' the defective
CFTR protein rather than actually correcting the mutant protein
itself. That being the case, in terms of potential treatments, the
specific pair of mutations carried in the CFTR genes of a patient
should not be relevant. These types of 'bypass' treatment could
theoretically be achieved by drugs that cause other proteins in the
cells of diseased organs to carry out the essential functions of the
CFTR protein. Alternative approaches involve actually replacing
the mutant CFTR protein either by introducing normal CFTR
protein into cells (protein therapy) or by inserting a normal copy
of the CFTR gene itself into cells (gene therapy). The technical
problems of achieving effective protein or gene therapy for CF are
currently the major obstacles to progress. If these can be overcome,
the chance of real treatment of CF is likely to be the same for all
patients, regardless of the mutations they have. We all hope that
these treatments will become available soon.

Genetic counselling and cystic fibrosis

The existence of prenatal and carrier detection tests has dramatically altered genetic counselling in CF. In the days before the location and discovery of the gene, most couples with an affected child made a conscious decision not to add further to the family. Options for such couples have now increased.

What is genetic counselling?

Genetic counselling is the provision of detailed information in an understandable form to individuals—most often couples of reproductive age—to help them make informed family planning decisions which comply with their own ethics as a couple.

The following are the facts which would be communicated to a couple with a CF affected child, during a counselling session.

(1) the nature of CF, its morbidity, prognosis, and burden for the baby and the family.

(2) the risk of having a further affected child, which is one in four in each pregnancy.

(3) the existence of accurate prenatal diagnostic tests by chorionic villus sampling at 10 weeks, with results available within a day or two. The risk of miscarrying from such a test is about 1 per cent above the pre-existing risk of any woman miscarrying after 10 weeks. The chance of miscarrying increases with age. One would advise a woman above the age of 35 to consider amniocentesis at 14 or 15 weeks rather than chorionic biopsy. For an extremely small number of couples, preimplantation diagnosis has allowed implantation of an early embryo conceived in a test-tube and shown to be free of CF.

In coming to a decision on adding to the family many factors will play a role. The severity of the disease as experienced by a particular couple is likely to influence their decision-making. Parents of young children with CF will often have been given very encouraging advice about what the future now holds in terms of improved prognosis and the hopes of new treatments. A nationally held register of couples who have had prenatal diagnosis has shown that young parents of young children with CF are less likely to have prenatal tests and terminate pregnancies than older parents of older children with CF, underlining the impression that when a disorder is seen or perceived to be serious, then couples will alter their reproductive behaviour, either by having no further children or by having tests in pregnancy with selective termination.

Couples base their reproductive decisions first on the procreative drive, which is both something internal and something imposed by family life and society. The existence of a significant risk of having a baby with a serious disorder, which may shorten life, will influence this drive.

For some people the existence of an accurate and safe prenatal test, particularly if available early in a pregnancy, will influence their decision. The same couple may view prenatal tests differently at different times of their lives: perhaps terminating one pregnancy, yet making a decision to continue with a second regardless of the outcome of a prenatal test.

With the prognosis in CF difficult to forecast accurately, it is not surprising that couples differ in their uptake of prenatal diagnosis. Paediatricians also differ in the emphasis which they may give to tests and termination of pregnancy as an option, while the CF clinic team of nurse, physiotherapist, and dietician also have views which may influence couples' decisions. We know one couple who wished to have tests in pregnancy with selective termination, but were worried that they would offend the paediatrician and his team who showed such devotion in the care of their beloved affected child. The availability of early tests like chorionic biopsy mean that couples have the option to keep the pregnancy private until results show an unaffected fetus.

People without an affected child who want genetic counselling

Adult men and women with CF may wish to have genetic counselling. Men are almost invariably sterile. However, although the male genital ducts are blocked or absent in CF, the testis does continue to function. Sperm have been obtained surgically by spiration from the ducts leading from the testis (the epididymis) see Figure 6). Unfortunately, it appears that when the affected man has the ΔF508 mutation in both CF genes or even when there s only one ΔF508 gene (with another mutation), the chances of a successful fertilization are reduced when compared to individuals with different mutations. Thus, hopes of fatherhood that are raised by this type of fertilization may be followed by disappointment after repeated unsuccessful attempts.

Women with CF would have a 1 in 44 chance of having an affected child themselves. Today one could test the partner—if he is negative for the commonest mutations in Britain which cover 85 per cent of CF genes, his risk of being a carrier would drop from 1 in 22 to 1 in 200 and their combined risk of an affected child would drop to 1 in 400. Of course the severity of the woman's CF and her ability to cope with a baby would dominate decisions on the wisdom of undertaking a pregnancy and would form part of the counselling session. Chorionic biopsy on an affected woman with a carrier partner has been safely performed, as has termination of an affected pregnancy.

More and more relatives of people with CF have been seeking genetic counselling with their partners. In the north-west of England the regional health authority has funded an 'active cascade' screening programme, based on known families or carriers discovered by other means. A nurse field worker makes contact with families with a history of CF or in which a carrier has been discovered, and offers simple CF screening tests to relatives and partners. These tests involve taking a mouthwash, which always then contains a few cells from the lining of the mouth, and analysis of the CF gene in these cells. The four commonest mutations are tested for, together with any particular mutation, no matter how rare, which is already known to be carried in the family. All relatives of people with CF have an increased chance of being carriers (see Table 2). Thus by testing in the family, one will occasionally find further carrier couples beyond the affected family with whom testing started. Of the first 1500 relatives or partners tested in this way at The Royal Manchester Children's Hospital, 15 such carrier couples have been detected, with their risk of having an affected child 1 in 4. The remainder have had their risks reduced with either

Table 2 Risk figures for various healthy relations, assuming a partner without a family history of CF

Relationship to person with CF	Before tests: Risk of being a carrier	Risk of CF in child
Parents	1 (100%)	1 in 4
Parent remarries	1 (100%)	1 in 100
Child of CF woman	1 (100%)	1 in 100
Brother or sister	2 in 3	1 in 150
Aunt or uncle	1 in 2	1 in 200
Grandparent	1 in 2	1 in 200
1st cousin	1 in 4	1 in 400
2nd cousin	1 in 8	1 in 800
3rd cousin	1 in 16	1 in 1600

Members of the general population without CF in the family have a 1 in 25 chance of being carriers. CF affects one in 2500 newborns.

Table 3 After tests which detect 88 per cent of CF genes

Results	Risk of having child with CF	Action
Both partners are carriers (rare)	1 in 4	Genetic counselling and tests offered in pregnancy
Relative carrier partner negative	1 in 836	Reassurance about low risk. Test offspring for CF if sickly
Relative negative partner carrier	1 in 1672	Retest to ensure no sample mix-up, reassure—low risk. Test child for CF if sickly
Relative negative partner negative	1 in 347 776 (tiny)	Strong reassurance

one or both partners being negative for CF mutations on testing. Many of the families with an affected individual have been very enthusiastic about contacting their relatives to advise them of the availability of tests. Tables 2 and 3 show risk figures for a hypothetical family and various relatives and partners before and after testing.

Population genetics and CF mutations

The ΔF508 mutation is present on about 70 per cent of CF chromosomes in northern Europe and North America. Analysis of the mutations in the CFTR gene that are carried by CF patients across Europe shows a gradient of distribution, moving south and east. The frequency of the ΔF508 mutation is much higher in Scandinavian countries, for example, than in Italy and Turkey.

As mutation analysis in the CF gene has progressed it has become clear that certain genetic populations have a high frequency of mutations that are much rarer in other populations. This is clearly of importance when devising CF screening strategies for different genetic groups.

Of particular note are the Ashkenazi Jewish population, who have a low frequency of the ΔF508 mutation but a much higher frequency of the two other mutations. In fact, by screening for these three mutations alone over 90 per cent of CF mutations can be detected in this population.

Other different mutations show a higher frequency in Italy, Northern Ireland, Germany, and Scandinavia.

Uncertain diagnosis of cystic fibrosis

It is not unusual for a diagnosis of possible CF to be made in cases where an individual does not have all the features of classical cystic fibrosis. The CFTR genes of many of these individuals have been analysed and some unusual new mutations in the CFTR gene have been found. In addition some individuals with what was formerly thought to be a completely different disease from CF, namely congenital absence of the vas deferens, have now been shown to carry mutations in both copies of their CFTR genes. It is probable that the clinical definition of cystic fibrosis may well have missed a percentage of patients who will remain undiagnosed in the absence of molecular analysis of their CFTR genes.

Frequency of CF

As has already been mentioned, CF is the most common potentially lethal autosomal recessive disease among Caucasians (white Indo-Europeans). The condition is extremely rare among Chinese races and in African Negroes. CF does occur in black Americans, natives of many Middle Eastern countries, and in Pakistan. In Caucasian races, however, the CF carrier frequency is about 1 in 22 to 25 individuals, and one baby in around 2000 to 2500 live births has the disease.

At present, we cannot explain the high frequency of CF particularly since 97 per cent of adult males with the disorder are sterile, and until very recently females with CF were not growing up to have children.

It should be mentioned that although in some diseases the likelihood of at-risk parents having an affected child is influenced by maternal age, birth order, or season of conception, none of these factors seems to have a role in CF. Cousin marriage does increase the likelihood of having a child with CF.

Mutation detection

The isolation of the CF gene in the autumn of 1989 opened up a completely new degree of accuracy in genetic counselling for the disease. Scientists can now look directly at the DNA in the CF gene in different individuals to search for defects. We know that about 70 per cent of people carrying a defective CF gene in England, northern European countries and North America all have the same lesion in their DNA. Three bases (see p. 80) are absent from the middle of their CF gene, which results in the loss of one amino acid building block from the protein that is coded for by the CF gene.

The loss of these three bases can be easily detected by a rather simple test.

The data from laboratories around the world on the frequency of mutations other than ∆F508 have generated a list of the 30 most common ones. Various tests are being developed that allow the detection of 5–12 of these mutations in the one assay. The precise mutations that need to be screened for will vary depending on the population that the CF patient comes from (see section on population genetics, p. 93). Even with these tests for multiple mutations there will remain certain mutations that will go undetected without substantial additional work. However, even without knowing the precise mutation carried by a CF family, genetic counselling can be given. These families are counselled on the basis either of linked DNA markers or by using polymorphic markers within the gene itself. Within the regions of the CFTR gene that do not code for the CFTR protein there are a number of blocks of repeated sequences. The precise number of repeats varies in different individuals but it is inherited stably on each parental chromosome. Hence these repeats provide a powerful tool for following inheritance of mutant CF chromosomes even in the absence of precise mutation information.

Once two parents are known to be carriers of CF, either due to the previous birth of an affected child or following direct genetic testing, they can be offered prenatal diagnosis of CF at future pregnancies.

Methods of prenatal diagnosis

The methods described below are currently used to diagnose a number of diseases before birth. Most methods of prenatal diagnosis rely on obtaining a small sample of material from, or produced by, the unborn child (the fetus). A biochemical test or a study of the chromosomes can then be carried out on this sample. This material may be a sample of amniotic fluid (the fluid surrounding the developing embryo, which contains many cell types that have been shed by the fetus and the membranes around it), a sample of the fetal blood taken from the umbilical cord, or a small piece of

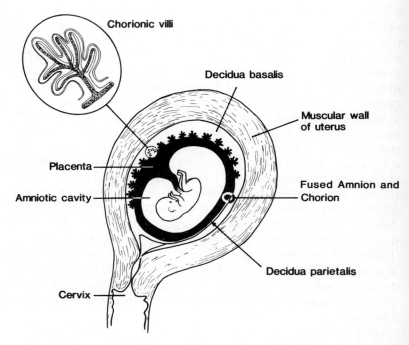

Figure 19 Diagram to show the human embryo in the amniotic sac about 12 weeks into pregnancy.

the rumpled outer surface of the membranes surrounding the fetus, known as chorionic villi (see Figure 19). All the procedures discussed have an acceptably low risk of interfering with the pregnancy, and have been used successfully in the prenatal diagnosis of a variety of different genetic diseases.

Amniocentesis

This test is usually carried out 16–18 weeks into the pregnancy. It involves collecting a small amount of amniotic fluid from around the fetus. It was the first technique developed for prenatal diagnosis of fetal abnormalities and is still the most frequently used. Following amniocentesis there is slightly less than one per cent increase in the chance of a miscarriage, and around a one per cent increase in the chance of a premature birth. Several tests can be carried out on this amniotic fluid. The fluid itself may have certain biochemical measurements carried out on it directly. For example, the level of a particular protein called alphafetoprotein that is present in amniotic fluid is characteristically found to be higher in defects of spine development such as spina bifida. There are also cells present in the amniotic fluid, and these may be grown (cultured) in the laboratory. The cultured cells can then be analysed to look for markers that are characteristic of particular diseases. One such marker is the number of chromosomes within each cell. Fetuses that have Down's syndrome (which often used to be known as mongolism), for example, carry three copies of chromosome 21 instead of the usual two.

Fetal blood sampling

This more recent technique involves taking a blood sample from the unborn child. The blood is most readily drawn from the vessels in the umbilical cord. The method has been used successfully in the prenatal diagnosis of thalassaemias (defects in the structure of haemoglobin, the molecule that carries oxygen around the blood system). The test is performed after about 18 weeks of pregnancy. It carries a small (1 per cent) risk of miscarriage.

Chorionic villus sampling

Amniocentesis and fetal blood sampling are only useful for diagnosis at a quite late stage of pregnancy (16–18 weeks). At such a late stage, termination of the pregnancy is very difficult for the mother, both physically and mentally. Chorionic villus sampling, however, can be carried out much earlier in the pregnancy (between 8 and 12 weeks after conception). The method involves the physical removal of a small piece of the rumpled outer surface (villi) of the membranes surrounding the fetus (the chorion). (Part of the chorion forms the placenta later in pregnancy, see Figure 19.) Rapid results can be obtained with chorionic villus sampling, because tests are carried out directly on the sample itself. This is in contrast to amniocentesis, where cells from the amniotic fluid usually must be grown in the laboratory until enough cells have been produced for testing. Hence chorionic villus sampling provides a method of early diagnosis of hereditary disorders. The risk factors associated with this procedure are nearly as low as those for amniocentesis. Allowing for the natural loss of about 4 per cent of fetuses between around 10 weeks' gestation and normal term, chorionic villus sampling increases this figure to around 6 per cent (in other words an added 2 per cent risk).

The basis of the procedure is to locate the position of the developing fetus and the chorionic tissue using ultrasound (see Figure 19). Solid objects deflect very high frequency sound waves (ultrasound) passed across the abdomen and these deflections are translated into an image of the developing pregnancy on a television screen. A thin, hollow tube is then passed through the cervix (the neck of the womb) and guided to the chorion using the image on the ultrasound scan. A very small piece of chorion (about 2 mm wide) is sucked into the tube and removed for testing. The sample may also be taken through the wall of the abdomen, similar to amniocentesis. Chorion tissue is growing very rapidly at this stage in pregnancy, so the cells in the sample will be dividing fast. This is ideal for rapid chromosome analysis, as well as for direct investigation using the techniques of biochemistry and molecular biology. The vast majority of prenatal diagnostic tests for CF are now carried out by chorionic villus sampling (CVS).

Ultrasound

As explained in the previous section, ultrasound can be used to obtain a picture of the developing pregnancy. This image on its own can be useful in showing up certain abnormalities in the unborn child. These are generally malformations of the fetus that alter its normal appearance in an ultrasound scan; for example, large-scale abnormalities of the spinal cord. Meconium ileus, the blockage of the bowel that occurs in some CF babies and was discussed in Chapter 3, may occasionally be detected by ultrasound scanning. Its role in the prenatal diagnosis of CF is a very limited one, but it may be useful in conjunction with other tests in suggest-

g that a fetus may have CF. Ultrasound has the advantage of
eing non-invasive and so does not increase the chance of spon-
neous miscarriage.

re-implantation testing for CF

is also possible to detect a genetic disease such as CF in the
rtilized embryo when it only contains a few cells and has not yet
nplanted into the womb. The test involves using the technique
at is already well-established in the treatment of infertility and is
nown as *in vitro* fertilization. This involves removing eggs from a
oman and fertilizing them with her partner's sperm in a test-tube.
he ensuing embryos are then placed back in the mother's womb to
nplant and develop into healthy babies.

In preimplantation diagnosis, one or sometimes two cells are
moved at the stage when all the cells of the embryo still have the
dividual capacity to grow into a fully formed baby. These two
ells are used to test whether the embryo has CF. The removal of
e two cells does not damage the rest of the cells in the embryo and
the test is safe. Preimplantation diagnosis is not widely available
s it requires highly specialized expertise. Those few couples who
re taken on to programmes of trying to achieve a pregnancy in this
ay have to be prepared for considerable disruption to their normal
utines. Both prospective parents need initial tests and counselling
r their individual suitability. If accepted the mother needs hor-
one treatment to ripen a number of eggs, then tests to determine
hen they are ripe; the ripe eggs are removed by laparoscopy
erformed by inserting a fine, flexible, fibreoptic tube into the
bdomen, inspecting the ovaries, and removing the ripest-looking
ggs). Five or six of the healthiest-looking eggs are then fertilized
ith the husband's sperm. After 48 hours, if fertilization has oc-
urred the healthiest looking embryos are selected and one or some-
mes two cells removed by micropipette from each. Tests for the
elevant CF mutations are then performed. In the earliest successful
xample, embryos with no CF genes were selected for reimplanta-
ion. Were such facilities to be freely available, there is no doubt
hat there are couples who would prefer this option to one of testing
1 pregnancy with the option of termination.

This group includes those who have had prenatal diagnosis in th past, which may have resulted in the abortion of an affected fetus those who by religious or moral conviction view preimplantation diagnosis as different to antenatal diagnosis during pregnancy; an couples who will not accept abortion.

Prenatal diagnostic tests for CF

It is now possible to offer the vast majority of couples at risk for CF a prenatal diagnostic test for the disease. The precise test offered will be a DNA-based test. In other words, it will be carried out on DNA extracted from fetal tissue (be it chorionic villi or single cells in the same way as tests are done on the DNA in the blood cells o the parents.

Further reading

Gosden, C., Nicolaides, K., and Whitting, V. (1994). *Is my baby all right? A guide for expectant parents*. Oxford University Press.

New treatments

There is still no cure for cystic fibrosis. However, gradual progress is being made in treating at least some aspects of the disease.

DNAse

The mucus in the lungs of CF patients is generally thicker and more sticky than normal. This is due at least in prt to the presence of DNA (the genetic material) from the cells, which are produced by the immune system of the body to combat lung infections. When these cells have performed their defence operation they die and the DNA they contain is released into the surrounding mucus. DNA is a tough, fibrous substance so it can increase the thickness of the mucus. Scientists have developed a means of producing large amounts of an enzyme that is able to digest and break down DNA. The enzyme is a natural human enzyme that has been inserted into bacteria by genetic engineering. The genetically modified bacteria are thus able to make the human DNAse enzyme. The DNAse converts thick CF mucus to a free-flowing substance. DNAse (marketed under the name of Dornase Alfa (Pulmozyme®)) has been subjected to extensive clinical trials in the UK and the USA, during which CF patients take a nebulized dose of DNAse once a day. It has generally been found to be effective and to have only side-effects such as hoarseness and sore throat in a few patients. It may not be effective for all CF patients. However, where it is a useful treatment it usually starts loosening mucus after the first dose, building up to noticeable breathing improvement after three or four days. The treatment has to be continuous since lung function generally returns to pretreatment levels three or four days after cessation of treatment. To date there is no evidence for any adverse long-term effects of DNAse treatment. Further, it is known that DNAse only digests DNA that is outside living cells so other tissues should not be damaged by the treatment.

As with most such 'genetically engineered' treatment products i
is expensive, though it should become widely available durin
1994.

Gene therapy

During the past year there has been a great deal of media coverag
of the proposed clinical trials of gene therapy for a number o
genetic diseases including cystic fibrosis. In this section we examin
what exactly gene therapy is; how it might work in the case of cysti
fibrosis; whether it is likely to work; and, if it works, on what time
scale.

What is gene therapy?

The principle of gene therapy is the straightforward idea that i
should be possible to correct the defect in a genetic disease by in
serting a normal copy of a gene into specific cells from the patient
The model can apply equally well for any genetic disease that i
caused by errors in a single gene. However, the theoretical likeli
hood that the approach will work will be largely dependent on th
accessibility of the cells that have to be corrected in order to cur
the disease. A good illustration of this problem is provided by com
paring a disease of the immune system with a disease of muscl
function. The cells of the body that comprise the immune system
are largely to be found in the bone marrow and in circulating cell
in the blood. This makes them relatively accessible for the insertio
of replacement genes. In contrast, trying to correct the genetic in
formation in muscle cells will be much more difficult as they canno
easily be reached.

How would gene therapy for CF be done?

Treatment of CF digestive disease is time-consuming and an annoy
ance, but by taking adequate pancreatic enzyme supplements th
digestive disease that is part of CF can be largely controlled. Thi
leaves the lungs as the main cause of severe illness in CF, hence, th
primary target for CF gene therapy is the layer of surface (epithelial

cells lining the lungs. Obviously this has certain advantages since the lungs are relatively accessible from outside the body. One could envisage inhalation of an aerosol spray as a means to deliver normal genes into the lung.

However, it is not quite as simple as this for a number of reasons. First, even though we know the precise structure of the CF gene and the protein that it codes for we know relatively little about what controls and regulates its functioning in the body; how much normal CFTR is needed to correct cells; and whether in order to cure CF lung disease, it would be necessary to target normal genes to the precise cells deep within the glands of the lung that are the only site where CFTR protein is found after birth.

Preliminary experiments attempting gene therapy in genetically engineered mice with cystic fibrosis suggest that at least in terms of correcting the failure to move salt out of epithelial cells, gene therapy of a number of cell types in the lung may be effective. Despite this encouraging data, it should be remembered that having the desired effect on a CF mouse lung is a very different achievement from curing the disease in the lungs of a person with CF. Mice with CF do not have lung disease comparable to that seen in humans with CF and it will be infinitely more difficult to achieve CF gene therapy in a diseased human CF lung with its characteristic problems of mucus accumulation and lung-tissue damage.

Potential risks of gene therapy

Another of the major hurdles that still has to be overcome prior to effective CF gene therapy is the establishment of a safe means of delivering the new CF gene into the cells of the lung. This presents problems because in order to make sure that sufficient CFTR protein is made from the introduced CF gene, scientists have designed pieces of DNA that use genetic signals from other species, including some segments of viral DNA to activate and control the CF gene. These segments of 'foreign' DNA are very well characterized and most efficient, probably much more so than the natural biological signals that regulate the CFTR gene. The whole gene therapy stratagem is dependent on the foreign genetic signals but clearly it is essential to minimize the risks of any protocols that are being used. Scientists must be sure, beyond reasonable doubt, that the segments of foreign DNA they are using will not have any unforeseen side-effects.

Another problem that has to be addressed is how to deliver the new gene into the cells, all of which are surrounded by a layer of lipid, the cell membrane. Some attempts at gene therapy have involved actually infecting the cells with the new piece of DNA by encapsulating it in modified viral 'carriers'. In these modified viruses there has been an attempt to remove the harmful portions of the virus and those parts that stimulate the body to produce antibodies directed against the virus. Two viruses, adenovirus and a much smaller adeno-associated virus, are being developed as potential gene therapy vehicles in the United States, Netherlands, and France. The type of adenovirus being modified is one of those that is often found in the human airways. Unfortunately, one of the first CF patients in the USA who was exposed to this means of gene therapy developed signs of inflammation in the respiratory system following the use of a modified adenovirus incorporating normal CFTR.

An alternative method is to attach the new gene to the surface of lipid (fatty) balls (called liposomes), that will naturally fuse with the lipid in the cell membrane of the cells that line the airways. This might prove to be the method of choice. A problem with the use of liposomes is that they are very inefficient when compared to the virus carriers, and that production costs for such a system may prove to be extremely high.

Another theoretical risk of gene therapy is that the new gene that has been inserted into the body of a CF patient may enter not only the cells to which it has been targeted in the airways. There is a tiny, theoretical chance that the new gene could find its way into the germ cells of the body, that is the eggs of the female or sperm of the male. This would imply that a treated, affected female could pass on the normal gene and any associated carrier DNA that she had received by gene therapy in addition to or instead of the mutant CF genes that she would have been biologically destined to transmit. (Remember, nearly all males with CF are sterile and hence this would not generally be a potential problem in males who had received gene therapy.) In Britain the ethics committee set up by the British government has ruled that gene therapy aimed at altering the germ-line is unethical. The first patients chosen for gene therapy in Britain have all been male, but it is likely that as soon as it is established that no normal gene has entered their germ-lines, females will also be entered in these trials.

Who grants permission for gene therapy experiments?

It will be reassuring to readers to know that in both the UK and North America, where CF gene-therapy experiments are being attempted, there are independent review committees that have to give permission for any such protocols to be carried out. These review committees include individuals from all walks of life including lawyers, ministers of religion, doctors, and philosophers, among others. Scientists and clinicians who are intending to carry out a gene-therapy trial have to compile extensive proposals detailing all aspects of the trial. This will include, in addition to the scientific protocols, particular attention to safety, clinical protocols, and trial design to ensure that the results that are obtained are significant.

What is the time scale for CF gene therapy?

At the time of writing, several CF gene therapy trials are now under way. However, they are all at an early stage and, quite properly, are progressing cautiously. Most of the trials involve carrying out local gene therapy on a very small part of the layer of epithelial cells that line the nose. This provides a means of assessing the efficiency of the system and of addressing the overriding safety aspects. The CF patients who are being offered the opportunity of entering these trials are generally adults, who are able to give their own informed consent. It is likely that the preliminary phases of the CF gene-therapy trials will take several years to complete as some relatively long-term issues have to be addressed. We should know within the next five years or so whether CF gene therapy is likely to be feasible. However, if it does work it is still likely to be many years before this becomes a proven means of treating the disease.

9 Organizations concerned with cystic fibrosis

(A1) The Cystic Fibrosis Research Trust

The Cystic Fibrosis (CF) Research Trust was founded in 1964 by the late John Panchaud, an international businessman whose daughter had CF. Together with Dr Archie Norman (Consultant Physician to John Panchaud's daughter) and Consultant Paediatrician Dr David Lawson, John Panchaud set up the CF Trust in part of his own offices in the City of London.

The objectives of the trust today are the same as they were when it was founded:

1. To finance research in order to find a complete cure for cystic fibrosis, and in the meantime, to improve current methods of treatment.
2. To form regions, branches, and groups throughout the United Kingdom, for the purpose of helping and advising parents about the everyday problems of caring for CF children.
3. To educate the public about the disease and, through wider knowledge, to help promote earlier diagnosis.

The trust raises funds continuously for CF research, through national events such as the annual 'CF week' and by the local activities of its regional groups and branches. In fact, since its foundation, the trust has provided over £15 million towards its objectives. A Research and Medical Advisory Committee, consisting of members of the medical and scientific community, advise on how the trust can best spend its resources.

The CF Trust's association with local groups is strong. It depends on regional branches and groups for the majority of its income; at the same time it acts as an information source for branches. The trust produces a valuable regional and branch group manual. This manual covers topics as wide-ranging as how to form and run the branch or group; the officers needed and how meetings should be organized; efficiency in fund-raising activities; publicity for the trust through local newspapers, radio, and television; and government grants available to CF patients and their families.

(A2) The North American Cystic Fibrosis Foundation [CFF]

The CFF was founded in 1955 to fund research into treatment and cure for CF and to improve the quality of life of individuals with the disease. It currently funds 11 multidisciplinary research centres and 9 gene therapy centres at universities and medical schools across North America. In addition to supporting basic research and clinical studies, the organization finances more than 120 CFF care centres which provide comprehensive care for those with CF.

The CFF produces brochures and fact sheets on many CF-related topics: for example, health insurance and financial assistance programmes. It also acts as an advocacy body to increase basic science funding and represent the interests of those with CF. The research, medical care, public policy, and education programmes of the CFF are financed by the fund-raising efforts of volunteers at 70 CFF branches and field offices across the USA.

The Canadian Cystic Fibrosis Foundation (CCFF) fulfils a similar role in Canada.

(B) Association of Cystic Fibrosis Adults (United Kingdom)

The aims and objectives of this association are:

1. To help the CF adult to lead as full and independent a life as possible.
2. To promote the exchange of information.
3. To act as a forum for improving the management of problems encountered by CF adults, both medical and otherwise.
4. To provide encouragement for all those with CF and CF families.

5. To assist wherever possible the efforts of the CF Research Trust.

There is now an active International Association of CF Adults (IACFA).

(C) The International Cystic Fibrosis (Mucoviscidosis) Association

The International Cystic Fibrosis (Mucoviscidosis) Association (ICF(M)A) was also founded in 1964, on the initiative of the American and Canadian CF Foundations. This organization is an international body, with one national association representing each country. In countries where there is not yet a national CF association, individuals are elected as associate members of the ICF(M)A to represent their countries until a national association has been formed and recognized by the ICF(M)A.

A Scientific and Medical Advisory Council (SMAC), composed of one medical or scientific member from each national association, meets once every four years. This meeting coincides with the major international CF conferences held under the auspices of the ICF(M)A, which bring together the majority of CF research scientists and physicians, a large number of CF allied professionals and lay people. In the intervals between CF congresses, a thirteen-member executive carries out the functions of the SMAC. This executive meets annually in parallel with the European Working Group for Cystic Fibrosis, which provides continuity in Europe between international meetings. In America the annual North American Cystic Fibrosis conference performs a similar function.

Together the ICF(M)A meetings have provided an international forum for the discussion of the personal, organizational, social, and technical problems of CF. Through this organization, the well-established associations have been able to provide help and guidance to new national associations in the process of setting up. This advice has always tried to take into account the different cultural environments operating in different countries. Key factors here are, for example, the level of involvement of the State in medical and social services and research facilities; variations in national wealth and economic priorities in health care; and attitudes to charities, their organizations, and fund-raising activities both within government and in the community at large.

Within these constraints the purposes of the ICF(M)A, in common with those of its affiliated national associations are as follows:

1. The furtherance of the interests of children and adults who have cystic fibrosis. The improvement of medical care available to these people and of the psychological and social care available to them and their families.
2. The stimulation, support, and advancement of research into the nature, cause, prevention, treatment, alleviation, and cure of cystic fibrosis.
3. The coordination of information services and the interchange of information on all phases of cystic fibrosis.
4. To assist in the formation of national associations devoted to cystic fibrosis, where they are required but do not yet exist.
5. The holding of meetings of representatives of government agencies, organizations, and individuals interested in the prevention, treatment, and cure of cystic fibrosis.

There are now some 33 countries whose national CF organizations are members of ICF(M)A and about nine others with associate membership. The full addresses of all these associations (correct as of June 1994) are given in Appendix 1.

Appendix 1: International Cystic Fibrosis (Mucoviscidosis) Association

Executive Committee

President Mr Martin Weibel, Fliederweg 45, CH-3138 Uetendorf, Switzerland.

Immediate Past President Mrs Inge Saxon-Mills, Olgiata 15, Isola 1/B, 00123 Rome, Italy.

Secretary Mrs Michelle Roche, 323 Lippens Avenue, Montreal, Quebec, Canada H2M 1H7.

Treasurer John Edkins FCA, Cystic Fibrosis Trust, Alexandra House, 5 Blyth Road, Bromley, Kent BR1 3RS, United Kingdom.

Vice President Mr Ian A. Thompson, McArthur Thompson & Law, P. O. Box 3598, Halifax, N S, Canada B3J 3J2.

Vice President Mr Per Espeli, Kommunenes Sentralforbund, Box 1378 Vika, 0114 Oslo, Norway.

World Health Organization Liaison Officer Liliane Heidet, 124 Chemin de la Montagne, CH-1224 Chene-Bougeries, Switzerland.

Members

Argentina Mrs M. L. Saporiti de Endler, Assoc Argentina de Lucha Contra La Enfermedad, Fibroquistica del Pancreas, Mansilla 2814, 3° piso Depto 14 Capital, 1425 Buenos Aires.

Australia Mrs Helen Griffiths, President, Australian Cysti Fibrosis Associations Federation, Macquarie Hospital Campu P. O. Box 254, North Ryde NSW 2113.

Austria Mr Wolfgang Dangl, Österreichische Gesellschaft zι Bekämpfung der Cystic Fibrose, Obere Augartenstraße 26 2ι A 1020 Wien.

Belgium Madame Annick Maréchal, Assoc Belge de Lutte contκ la Mucoviscidose, Avenue Borle Laan 12, 1160 Bruxelles.

Brazil Mr Gustavo B. Eboli, Associacao Brasileira de Assoc Mucoviscidose, Hospital de Clinicas de P Alegre, C P # 508ι 90041 970 Porto Alegre RS.

Bulgaria Cystic Fibrosis Assoc of Bulgaria, Research Institute (Paediatrics, Medical Academy, D Nesterov str II, 1606 Sofia.

Canada Mrs Cathleen Morrison, Executive Director, Canadiι Cystic Fibrosis Foundation, 2221 Yonge Street Suite 601, Torontc Ontario, M4S 2B4.

Chile Mr Patricio Lira, Corp para la Fibrosis Quistica dι Pancreas, La Canada 6505 (i), La Reina, Santiago.

Colombia Dr Jorge Enrique Palacios R M D, Liga Colombian Contra la Fibrosis Quistica LAFCOL, Hospital San Juan de Dio: Calle 20N, 4N 45 Consultorio 202, Cali.

Costa Rica Dra Reina Gonzalez, Asociacion Costaricense ժ Fibrosis Quistica, Apdo 337 1200, Zona 9, Pavas, San Jose.

Cuba Prof Manuel Rojo Concepción, Comisión Cubana ժ Fibrosis Quistica, Hospital Pediátrico Juan Manuel Márquez, Aν 31 esq 76 Zona Postal 14, Municipio Marianao, Ciudad Habanι Código Postal 1400.

Czech Republic Mrs Helena Holubová, The Club of Parents and Friends of Children with Cystic Fibrosis, Bitouská 1226/7, 140 00 Praha 4.

Denmark Mrs Hanne Wendel Tybkjaer, Danish Cystic Fibrosis Association, Hyrdebakken 246, DK-8800 Viborg.

France Monsieur Hervé Garrault, General Manager, Association française de Lutte contre la Mucoviscidose, 76 rue Bobillot, 75013 Paris.

Greece Z. Papavassilopoulou, General Secretary, Hellenic Cystic Fibrosis Assoc, Angelou Sikelaniou 8, Neo Psychico, Athens 5452.

Hungary Dr Klara Holics, President, CF Foundation, H-1124 Ürök u 15, Budapest.

Iceland Mr Hördur Bergsteinsson, Cystic Fibrosis Assoc of Iceland, Barnaspitali Hringsins, Landspitalinn v/Baronsstig, 101 Reyjavik.

Israel Mr Ami Kolumbus, Israel Cystic Fibrosis Assoc, 5 Benyamini Street, Tel Aviv.

Italy Lega Italiana Delle Assiazioni per la Lotta contra la Fibrosi Cistic, c/o Ospedale Civile Maggiore, Piazzali A Stefani 1, 37126 Verona.

Mexico Dr José Luis Lezana, Medical Director, Asociación Mexicana de Fibrosis Quistica AC, Altavista # 21 CP 01000, Col San Angel, Mexico D.F.

Netherlands Mr Herman J. Weggen, Nederlandse Cystic Fibrosis Stichting, Lt Gen van Heutszlaan 6, 3743 JN Baarn.

New Zealand Mr Bruce Dunstan, General Manager, Cystic Fibrosis Assoc of New Zealand, 187 Cashel St, P. O. Box 22776, Christchurch 1.

Norway Ms Reidun Jahnsen, President, Norsk Forening f∢ Cystisk Fibrose, Postboks 114, Kjelsås, 0411 Oslo 4.

Poland Mr Stanislav Sitko, Polish Society Against Cystic Fibrosi⟩ os Tysiaclecia 62/64, Krakow.

Portugal Dr M. Celeste Barretto, Associacao Portuguesa ⟨ Fibrose Quistica, Apartado Nr 9824, 1911 Lisboa.

Republic of Ireland Mrs Bridie Maguire, Cystic Fibrosis Asso⟨ of Ireland, CF House, 24 Lower Rathmines Road, Rathmine⟩ Dublin 6.

Romania Professor dr Ioan Popa, President, Romanian C Association, Str Paltinis nr 1–3, 1900 Timisoara.

South Africa Mr Alain Woolf, National CF Association, 25 Ho⟩ Road, Orange Grove 2192.

Spain Mr Andrès Casanova, Federacion Espanola de Fibros⟩ Quistica, c/Lladro y malli 10, 46007 Valencia.

Sweden Mrs Brigitta Hellquist, Swedish Cystic Fibrosis Assoc ation, Box 1827, 751 48 Uppsala.

Switzerland Mrs Regula Salm Müller, Schweizerische Gesellscha für Cystische Fibrose (Mucoviscidose), Bellevuestraße 166, 309 Spiegel/Bern.

United Kingdom John Edkins Esq, Cystic Fibrosis Trus⟩ Alexandra House, 5 Blyth Road, Bromley, Kent BR1 3RS.

USA Dr Robert Beall, Cystic Fibrosis Foundation, 6931 Arlingto⟨ Road Suite 200, Bethesda, Maryland 20814.

Uruguay Mr Enrique Silver, Asociacion de Fibrosis, Quistica d∢ Uruguay, Francisco Rodrigo 2975, aptdo 4 11, 600 Montevideo

Associate Members

El Salvador   Fundaccion para la Fibrosis Quistica de El Salvador, Res Bethania, Pje 4, No 14-e, Santa Tecla.

Estonia   Dr Tlina Klaassen, President, Estorian Cystic Fibrosis Society, Tartu University, Inst of Molecular and Cell Biology, 2 Jakobi St Tartu EE2400.

Egypt   Prof. Dr Ekram Abdel-Salam, Cystic Fibrosis Association, 11 Falaki Square, Cairo 11111.

Finland   Ms Leena Jokinen, Secretary, Hoikan Kuntoutuskeskus, 38100 Karkku.

Pakistan   Dr Tasleem Akhtar, Research Director, PMRC Research Centre, Khyber Medical College, Peshawar.

Russia   Dr Tatiana E. Gembitzkaya, Chief of CF Centre, Institute of Pulmonology, Roentgen st 12, 197089 St Petersburg.

Saudi Arabia   Dre Hisham Nazer FRCP, Professor of Paediatrics, King Faisal Specialist Hospital and Research Centre, P.O. Box 3354, Riyadh 11211.

Turkey   Dr Ayhan Göçmen MD, Professor of Paediatrics, Institute of Child Health, Hacettepe University, Hacettepe/Ankara.

Venezuela   Dra Julieta Conde Di Mase, Fibrosis Quistica de Venezuela AC, Calle Los Abogados Av, Facultad con Av, Las Ciencias Quinta Montecarlo, Los Chaguaramos, Caracas 1041.

Appendix 2: Glossary

acidosis — condition resulting from accumulation of acid o depletion of the alkaline (bicarbonate) reserves in the blood or body tissues.

aerosols — medications given by inhalation, usually involving the wearing of a mask over the nose and mouth. In CF antibiotics bronchodilators, saline, and occasionally mucolytics are given thi way.

alleles — the two forms of the same gene coexisting in the same cell one being inherited from each of the parents.

alveoli — tiny, air-filled sacs in the lung tissue.

artificial insemination by donor — insemination of a woman with sperm from an unknown donor in a sperm bank instead of that of her partner.

aspergillosis — inflammatory reaction to infection by the fungus *Aspergillus fumigatus*.

autosome — all chromosomes other than the sex chromosomes.

bacteria — microorganisms (e.g. *Staphylococcus*, *Pseudomonas*), some of which may invade healthy tissues, others only damaged tissue, to cause infections. Some bacteria, e.g. the *Bacillus coli* of the large bowel, cause no infection and are in fact necessary for health.

ball-valve effects — these occur in those segments of the lung that have become overdistended through air getting past an obstruction on breathing in, but less getting past on breathing out.

base — a substance that reacts with an acid to form a salt and water only.

bronchiectasis — a state of permanent weakening of the bronchial walls, often because of infections and ball-valve phenomena which result in poor drainage of infected mucus.

bronchioles — small bronchi.

bronchodilator — a substance capable of relieving bronchospasm.

bronchospasm — a reversible spasm (contraction) of the bronchi.

bronchus (plural **bronchi**) — major branch of the airways.

carrier — an individual who has inherited a particular defective form of a recessive gene from one of his parents, but a normal form from the other. He thus 'carries' the defective gene, but suffers no ill effects from it.

cholecystitis — inflammation of the gall bladder, often associated with gallstones.

chromosomes — the structures within each cell that contain the genetic material.

cilia — minute mobile, hair-like processes projecting from the outer surface of a cell. The airways are lined with ciliated cells.

cirrhosis — fibrosis of the liver, interfering with the passage of blood from the intestine through liver cells.

coeliac disease — an inability to digest wheat proteins.

consanguinity — inbreeding between genetically related members of the same family.

cystic fibrosis transmembrane conductance regulator (CFTR) — the protein made by the CF gene. It is thought to regulate movements of charged molecules across cell membranes.

ΔF508 — the common mutation found in 70 per cent of CF genes in northern Europe and North America. It is caused by the loss of three bases in the DNA resulting in the absence of the amino acid phenylalanine at position 508 in the protein.

diploid — cells carrying two sets of genetic information.

diuretic — substance causing the increased production of urine.

DNA (deoxyribonucleic acid) — the major component of the genetic material. The biological molecule that codes for all the information needed to construct a human being from a single fertilized egg.

DNA amplification — a technique for making many thousands of copies of a specific piece of DNA.

dominant — a gene, the effects of which are not masked by the presence of its normal counterpart in the same cell.

duodenal intubation — a process whereby the end of a soft polythene tube is swallowed and passed via the stomach into the duodenum, allowing the contents to be studied chemically, both as regards enzymes and alkalinity.

emphysema — permanent overdistension of the alveoli in the lung.

endocrine glands — these pass their secretions directly into the bloodstream, e.g. insulin and glucagon from the pancreas.

enema — injection of liquid into the rectum.

erythrocytes — red blood cells, the cells that are responsible for carrying oxygen in the blood and so round the body.

exocrine gland — a gland that passes its secretions by ducts, e.g. trypsin and lipase from the pancreas. (The pancreas is both an exocrine and an endocrine gland.)

fibrosis — the replacement of normal tissue with scar tissue, e.g. in the pancreas. Hence the name *cystic fibrosis*: fluid-filled cysts develop in the obstructed parts of the pancreas.

flatus — breaking of wind.

genes — coding regions of DNA.

genome — all the genetic information of an individual.

haematemesis — the vomiting of blood. In CF this would most often be associated with cirrhosis and varices.

haemoptysis — the coughing of blood, usually indicative of advanced CF.

haploid — cells carrying one set of genetic information (i.e. eggs and sperm).

heart–lung transplants — replacement of heart and lungs of CF patient with those of an organ donor.

heterozygote — an individual who has inherited different forms of a particular gene from both parents.

homozygote — an individual who has inherited identical forms of a particular gene from both parents.

hormones — specific substances produced in endocrine glands (see above) that are secreted into the blood and are carried to all parts of the body. Hormones are quick-acting, required in very small amounts, and have a wide range of effects on body biochemistry.

ileus — literally, a disorder of motility of the ileum, resulting in the contents not being propelled towards the colon. In meconium ileus, contents are not propelled because of the tenacious meconium.

ileostomy — the bringing of a loop of ileum to open on to the anterior abdominal wall to allow bowel contents to be passed, when there is an obstruction lower down.

immunosuppressant drugs — drugs that suppress the natural immunological response of the body to reject foreign tissues and proteins.

intussusception — a pathological process in which a section of the small intestine folds into the adjoining region of downstream bowel, endangering its blood supply.

in vitro **fertilization** — fertilization of an egg by a sperm in a test-tube in the laboratory.

ion — an electrically charged atom or molecule.

isotonic — having the same electrolytic composition, as do most body tissues.

lingula — part of the upper lobe of the left lung.

malabsorption — inability to absorb food normally in intestines due to poor digestion.

MCT oil — oil containing medium-chain triglycerides. These can be absorbed directly into the bloodstream from the intestine.

meconium — the first dark-green stools of the newborn.

meconium ileus — an obstruction of the small intestine at birth.

meiosis — the cell division process by which haploid cells are made from diploid ones.

mesentery — the membrane carrying the blood vessels to and from the bowel.

messenger RNA — copied from DNA by transcription, this molecule is the blueprint for translation of the genetic information into biologically useful molecules, proteins.

mucolytic — substance capable of thinning mucus. It may do this by increasing the water content of the mucus or by breaking chemical bonds between sulphur and hydrogen.

mutation — the occurrence of a spontaneous abnormality in a gene that is not found in the genes of the parent's cells.

nasal polyp — a growth resulting from the heaping up of mucous membrane in the nostril. Common in older children with CF.

organ rejection — loss of function of donor organs due to the new host's immunological response to them.

osteomyelitis — infection of the bone, often caused by *Staphylococcus* bacteria, generally in people free of CF.

pancreatin — extract of animal pancreas.

parenteral — given by a route other than the alimentary canal (digestive system) — usually by vein.

pathogenesis — the evolution of the abnormal (pathological) changes of a disease process.

peritoneum — the membrane lining the walls of the abdomen.

peritonitis — an acute inflammation of the peritoneum.

phenylketonuria — a genetic disease that results in inability to break down phenylalanine in the diet.

pneumothorax — air trapped between the outside (pleural) surface of the lung and the chest wall. This splints the lung and prevents its normal movement during breathing. In CF it would occur with the rupture of overdistended (emphysematous) alveoli. Removal of the air by a needle attached to an underwater drain may be necessary.

probe — a segment of DNA that is complementary to part or all of the DNA sequence of interest.

prolapsed rectum — found in young infants with CF, usually before diagnosis. Malabsorption of fat, with very frequent stools, results in the inner linng of the rectum protruding through the anus.

proximal bowel — section of bowel closer to the mouth. (**Distal bowel** — bowel section further from mouth, i.e. closer to anus.)

recessive — a gene, the effects of which are masked by the presence of its normal counterpart in the same cell.

recombination — the physical process by which new combinations of genes are made by shuffling of the genetic information prior to cell division.

sclerosing agents — drugs that strengthen the blood vessel wall.

spirometer — an instrument for measuring the air breathed into and out of the lungs.

sputum — phlegm coughed up from the airway passages.

steatorrhoea — literally, fatty diarrhoea. Recognized by pale, bulky, foul-smelling stools.

steroids — a group of substances that can be natural or artificial and which have a wide range of effects when given as medicines, including suppression of immunological responses.

varices — dilated veins.

X-linked — a gene on the X chromosome.

Index